T
REALLY USEFUL
MEDITATION BOOK

THE
REALLY USEFUL
MEDITATION BOOK

LORRAINE CAVANAGH

Hodder & Stoughton

First published in Great Britain 1995

10 9 8 7 6 5 4 3 2 1

British Library Cataloguing in Publication Data
A record for this book is available from the British Library

ISBN 0 340 64186 X

Printed and bound in Great Britain by
Cox & Wyman Ltd, Reading, Berks
Typeset by Hewer Text Composition Services, Edinburgh

Hodder and Stoughton Ltd
A Division of Hodder Headline PLC
338 Euston Road
London NW1 3BH

For Sean, Meara and Alys

FOREWORD

There are many books around which try to adapt the Christian life to the modern world. They fail. They must. It is the strength of this book that it attempts just the opposite: an adaptation of ourselves to the true life of the spirit and the imagination. It straightens, I believe, the path to true wisdom, to lasting refreshment and an increasing appetite for self-awareness which allows positive action and lasting change. Not the least of these changes is to see ourselves as part of the human race and the whole of creation, not just as members of a Christian family.

I have long been an advocate of what T.S. Eliot called 'necessary idleness' to replace a superficial 'catch-phrase Christianity' with the stillness in which one can find true spiritual discernment. Here is a way, and one which seems to me uniquely fitted to Marthas or Marys of either sex. It is a book which will deepen as the reader deepens, and offer new insights year after year. It is, in short, a book for those who prefer life to that crass modern substitute lifestyle.

Nigel Forde
YORK 1995

CONTENTS

Acknowledgments

I should like to thank the following for permission to reproduce extracts from the publications detailed:

The Complete Book of Furniture Repair and Refinishing, R.P. Kenny (Peter Owen Publishers, London) for the recipe for Furniture Polish on p. 147;

The Creative Book of Party Decorations, Suzie Major (Salamander Books Ltd, London) for the Santa Face on p. 7, and Box (adapted) on p. 294;

The Complete Jewish Cookbook, Anne London and Bertha Kahn Bishov (proprietors: World Publishing Company) for three recipes: *Latkes* on p. 28, *Charoses* on p. 179, and Blintzes on p. 230;

Festive Crafts, Mary Ann Green (Random House UK Ltd, London) for the Floating Candles on p. 54;

The Bread Book, Martha Rose Shulman (Macmillan, London) for the Barley Bannocks on p. 132;

The Scented Room, Barbara Ohrbach (Sidgwick & Jackson, London) for the recipe for Rose Water on p. 168;

The Cookery Year (The Reader's Digest Association Ltd, London) for the Decorated Easter Eggs on p. 191;

The Church News Service for the story and illustration on p. 205, told by Joan Matthews of Whiston, Merseyside, in the CNS;

Wild Food, Roger Phillips (Pan Books Ltd, London) for the recipe for Elderflower Champagne on p. 210;

Chocolates, Sweets and Toffees, Jan Morgan (Cassell PLC, London) for three recipes: Sugared Almonds on p. 237, Fudge on p. 292, and Toffee Apples on p. 300;

Japanese Cookery, Peter and Joan Martin (Andre Deutsch Ltd, London, 1970) for the Japanese Salad on p. 254;

A Chain of Love, Kathryn Spink (SPCK, London) for the extract on p. 253;

Waiting on God, Simone Weil (Routledge and Kegan Paul) for the extract on p. 278;

Confessions, Saint Augustine, tr. R.S. Pine-Coffin (Penguin Classics, 1961) for the extract on p. 280;

The Book of Common Prayer for use in The Church in Wales, vol. 1 (The Board of Mission, Church in Wales Centre, Penarth) for extracts on pp. 3, 14, 34, and 297;

The Celtic Vision – Selections from the Carmina Gadelica, ed. Esther de Waal (St Bede's Publications, Petersham, Mass.) for the extract on p. 232; and

The Rule of St Benedict, tr. Abbot Parry OSB (Fowler Wright Books, UK) for the extract on p. 125.

I am also grateful to the following for their contributions and practical help: Jenny Balfourpaul, Chris Cooper, Sister Lisbeth CHN and Gladys Young.

Note

The readings follow the Christian Church's year. You will not necessarily cover all fifty-seven weeks, since the length of Trinitytide depends on when Easter falls and, as four Sundays are required for Advent, there will sometimes be fewer than twenty-six Sundays after Trinity Sunday. The feasts and Saints' days have been fitted generally into the overall fifty-six week scheme, with a few additions of my own, but the calendar year may not always tally precisely with the liturgical year outlined in the book. Please feel that you can use individual readings, meditations and recipes at any time of the year.

Most of the readings have been selected from the Alternative Service Book, the Welsh Book of Common Prayer, and from the readings appointed for the Roman Catholic Mass and the Orthodox Liturgy of the day. I have used the Revised Standard Version (RSV) of the Bible, which has always been my personal preference, because of the beauty of its language, but have also used the New Revised Standard Version (NRSV) where there is a danger of this language becoming exclusive.

PREFACE

This book came to be written out of a desire to bring Christian contemplative prayer within reach of those living busy lives in the modern world. Its chief purpose is to help readers to reach a point where their prayer becomes an integral part of daily living. Ideally, the two should be indistinguishable. The book began as a series of weekly meditations which appeared in our parish magazine. They were designed to help people to stay with the readings and collects prescribed for Sundays while they went about their normal weekday lives and this remains the first objective for *The Really Useful Meditation Book*. I hope that it will help to bring Christian contemplative prayer within easy reach of anyone, regardless of experience or lifestyle. It is not a book which sets out to evangelise, but in writing it I have particularly tried to address the situations and life problems faced by people who belong to no specific church or denomination and yet feel themselves to be Christians. I was in this predicament myself for many years, so am particularly sympathetic to their problems.

I am also concerned that those who have already begun to meditate on their own, or to pray in groups, should find in this book ways of developing their relationships with God and of seeing themselves as an integral part of his intricate and delicate scheme of life. I hope that anyone who uses the book, and certainly anyone who works through it for a year, will feel themselves to be more connected with the world and yet increasingly detached from its preoccupations and coldly materialistic values – more *in* the world and less *of* the world.

It is important to realise that we belong to each other as a human family, of which Christ came to be a part, and to all created beings, whether animal or plant, earth or sea, as well as to the sky and the elements. I am not calling for a pantheistic understanding of the Christian faith, only for the humility to listen to what those of a different denomination, a different faith or no faith at all, may have to teach us. We should also listen for the wisdom which God's Spirit may be trying to give us through the mysterious and beautiful planet which we have inherited and for which we are not only responsible to God, its creator, but to future generations. (These ideas are seldom alluded to directly, but it may be helpful to bear them in mind as you read and ponder the contents of this book.) I hope it will be a means of opening new doors and forging new paths for the intellect as well as the spirit.

The narrowness of the denominational corridors in which we find ourselves stifles natural human love and distorts the great truth which we all share. We could go a long way towards breaking down these constraints if we were to acquire the habit of thinking of ourselves as belonging to a single diverse family, something we take for granted but seldom put into practice. In order to assist this process, I have included a few Jewish feasts and customs, as the spiritual roots of all Christians lie in Judaism, whose beautiful prayers and ancient traditions still have much to teach us.

In compiling the book I have followed the Christian Church's liturgical year, because I believe it to be a most eloquent expression of the way in which the whole of creation and the understanding of the meaning of existence are Christ-centred and of his deigning to be born in what was the equivalent of a draughty shed in a hotel car park.

The Really Useful Meditation Book is designed to be used at any time of year. It has no beginning and no end and I hope will prove just as useful if it is begun in Lent as it would on the first Sunday in Advent.

Lorraine Cavanagh
February 1995

INTRODUCTION

Before embarking on any of these meditations you should try to get into a state of mind and body which is as relaxed as possible, although if you are a person who finds it difficult to relax under any circumstances don't feel that you are somehow 'not doing it right'. God can work with those who are stressed, anxious, or depressed, as easily as with the most experienced and recollected of contemplatives – and perhaps better. Nevertheless, for your own enjoyment and sense of well-being, here is a short exercise to do before you begin prayer. Spend five to ten minutes on it, depending on your own temperament and on the time available to you.

Spend a few minutes relaxing both inwardly and outwardly. Be physically aware, from the crown of your head to the tip of your toes. Relax the muscles of your face, neck, shoulders and hands. Feel the weight of your body centred from the top of your head, through your spine, to whatever you are sitting on. If you are sitting on a chair, be aware of your feet squarely on the floor. Let go of tension and of all the preoccupations, trivial or not, which fill your mind. If you find this difficult, don't try to drive them out. Just accept them and leave them to themselves, like noisy children playing in the room next door. In the same way, acknowledge, accept and let go of any outside noises or distractions which are beyond your control – traffic noise, for example.

Allow your breathing to become steady, but don't become too conscious of it. If thinking about breathing makes you breathless or dizzy, don't do this part of the exercise. Once your breathing is regular and peaceful, forget about your breathing pattern altogether.

When reading the passage of scripture or the meditation, be attentive to it from the heart, desiring that God's Spirit speak to you in it. Don't force yourself to concentrate and if you fall asleep, wake to a feeling of gratitude rather than guilt. If you have time, go back to wherever you left off.

ADVENT

First Sunday in Advent

Reading

Almighty God, give us grace that we may cast away the works of darkness, and put upon us the armour of light, now in the time of this mortal life, in which thy Son Jesus Christ came to visit us in great humility; that in the last day, when he shall come again in his glorious Majesty, to judge both the quick and the dead, we may rise to the life immortal; through him who lives and reigns with thee and the Holy Ghost, now and ever. Amen.

Collect

Meditation

A time of travelling from darkness to light, hastening as it does towards the winter solstice when the days will begin to grow imperceptibly longer. A time of promise and transformation, of being open to the impossible happening in ourselves, in our relationships, in our world. A time of hope. As we cast off the ways of darkness in preparation for the coming of the light and begin to think of presents and Christmas decorations with which to celebrate the love we have for one another and the love for the place which we call home, we look into our hearts at those attitudes, opinions and habits which need transforming.

Action

Here is a simple way to make your own Christmas wrapping paper. The bright colours will be a reminder of the joy that is soon to come into the world.

MARBLED PAPER

You will need:

Some lining paper or inferior quality computer paper, the flimsier the better. It must not be shiny.
1 small box of powdered size (easily available in art supply and DIY shops)
A large tray 2½cm or 5cm (1in or 2in) deep (a baking tray or photographic tray will do)
A selection of artists' oil paints
Turpentine or turpentine substitute (white spirit)
An old comb, skewer or nail

Bring 1½ litres (2 pints) of water to the boil and sprinkle the size powder into it, one tablespoon at a time, while stirring. Keep doing this until your fingers feel slightly slimy or sticky when you dip them lightly into the mixture. Thin the oil paint with turps or white spirit and drop the colours into the size mixture so that they form pools. If the colours disappear into the liquid, the mixture is too thin; if they turn into a lump, it is too thick. Drop different colours into each other and swirl them about using a comb or skewer. Gently lower the paper on to the surface and remove almost immediately. Dry flat. The paper can be ironed later on the reverse side using a very cool iron.

Saint Nicholas
6 December

Reading

I therefore, a prisoner for the Lord, beg you to lead a life worthy of the calling to which you have been called, with all lowliness and meekness, with patience, forbearing one another in love, eager to maintain the unity of the Spirit in the bond of peace (Eph. 4:1–3).

From the readings chosen for the Orthodox Liturgy on the feast of Saint Nicholas the wonderworker

Meditation

Saint Nicholas is honoured as the original Santa Claus. He was Bishop of Myra in the fourth century and wealthy in his own right. According to legend, he acquired his reputation for munificence by coming to the rescue of a poor man who had no dowries for his three daughters, so that the girls were unable to find good husbands. Saint Nicholas took a bag of gold one night and threw it through the window (it is also said, down the chimney) of the girls' bedroom, thereby assuring them of husbands and a secure future.

He is also remembered as the patron saint of prisoners and pawnbrokers. The three bags of gold are the basis for the pawnbroker's sign of three golden balls. The saint is also known to have campaigned vociferously for the release of prisoners, to the point of forcibly releasing them himself.

Christ comes to visit us in the prison which we have made for ourselves when we are tethered to the world's artificial values and priorities. The Christ-child waits to welcome us into his simplicity. The freedom and wealth which he offers us is the freedom to be the true 'selves' which we were created to be, rather than the people we have been conditioned to believe we are. Dare to own those real selves, forgiving whatever is shameful. Allow them to be, and allow the Christ-child in the poverty of his surroundings to love and welcome them as his own.

Action

Be a Santa Claus: perhaps by making a contribution to one of the many charities which care for those who have nowhere to go at Christmas, or by releasing someone from a debt or obligation. Affirm someone in their effort to break out of a mould or stereotype. If you have teenagers or young adults in your household, set aside your own role as parent or authority figure and give them a chance to respond to you as a person.

Celebrate Saint Nicholas and all those who are generous with their wealth. Here is a quick and easy way to make Santa faces to hang on the Christmas tree:

You will need:

   Scissors, glue, cardboard, coloured felt and sequins or small buttons.

Cut out the pieces in felt using the pattern on page 7.
Glue the main face section to a piece of cardboard, and when it is dry, cut around it.
Glue the other pieces, beginning with the nose and cheeks and ending with the moustache, which goes on top, and with a small circle on top of the pointed hat.
Place a loop of thread under the circle on top of the hat to hang up the face.
Glue on two sequins or small buttons for the eyes.

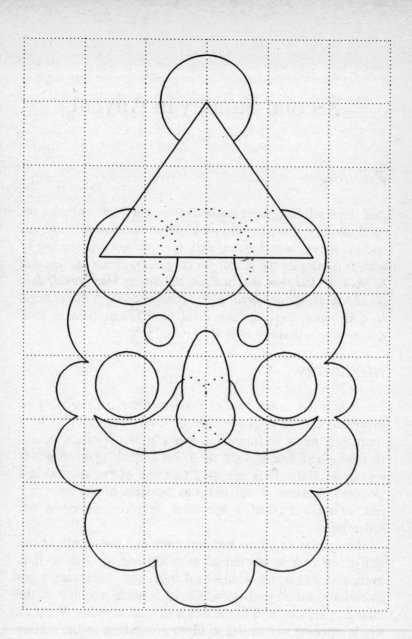

Second Sunday in Advent

Reading

And there will be signs in sun and moon and stars, and upon the earth distress of nations in perplexity at the roaring of the sea and the waves, men fainting with fear and with foreboding of what is coming on the world; for the powers of the heavens will be shaken. And then they will see the Son of man coming in a cloud with power and great glory. Now when these things begin to take place, look up and raise your heads, because your redemption is drawing near (Luke 21:25–8).

Meditation

Nowadays the words 'son of man' would most probably be expressed as 'one of the people' or 'ordinary person'. Christ frequently refers to himself in this way but reminds us also to look ahead and to look up to his coming again in power and great glory. It is tempting to think of the natural and political disasters of our times as portents of the last days, but we are not asked to speculate, only to look up to our redemption.

The coming of Christ happens over and over again in our daily lives and we should be as ready and as open to it in every moment as we would be if overnight there were 'signs in sun and moon and stars'. Christ is made manifest in the changing seasons and in the dawn of each new day. We look up, in opening our hearts to those around us, to the quality of the winter afternoon light, to the smell of good things cooking, and experience the Son of man – the man of the people, present to our present predicament, buying our lives back from emptiness and futility.

Action

The second Sunday in Advent is also kept by many Churches as Bible Sunday. So take time today, not only to read the Bible, but to adopt a plan for reading it throughout the coming year. We open our hearts to God in listening inwardly to his word. Most Christian bookshops have a wide selection of aids to Bible reading, ranging from vast commentaries to slim paperbacks which focus on one aspect or book of scripture and small booklets with a page and a single passage for each day.

Saint Lucy
13 December

Reading

Maidens shall follow in her retinue into the king's presence; all rejoicing, all triumph, those companions of hers, as they enter the palace of their Lord and King.

Gradual for the Mass

Meditation

The precise dating of Christ's birth is still a matter for conjecture. There are some who seek to justify the hijacking of Advent and Christmas by commercial interests with the argument that Jesus was probably born in September and that Christmas was used as a means of civilising the pagan winter festivities. But the true light that has come into the world is not so easily hidden. Just as Christ came at a point in history when all seemed lost for the Jewish people, who were once again under occupation, so he comes to the world year after year, in order to be with us in the dark winter months which lie ahead. The reality of the Incarnate Son of God is one of staggering simplicity. It is quite beyond rational comprehension but it is there all the same for those who are disposed to receive it. The child who is fully present to us in times of sickness, loneliness and anxiety offers us rest and distraction from the world. (Prayer is the enduring delight of play and conversation with the Christ-child. It is wisdom of God in the secret place of our inner being.)

Saint Lucy is thought of as the bearer of light. She was

martyred during the reign of the Emperor Diocletian in AD 304 for refusing to sacrifice to pagan gods and for refusing to break her vow of chastity in order to marry a non-Christian. It is said that her persecutors tried to drag her to a brothel, but even though she was only a young girl, she proved to be so heavy that three or four men were unable to move her. According to legend, her eyes were gouged out, but she was instantly and miraculously awarded a new pair.

Saint Lucy's feast day coincides with the darkest time of year and is particularly popular in Sweden where it marks the vernal equinox and the beginning of the pre-Christmas party season. She is commemorated in Swedish households with the baking of Lucy bread, or Lucy buns, which takes place the previous night.

Early on the morning of the 13th, long before dawn, the youngest girl of the household is dressed in white with a red sash around her waist. She is crowned with a garland of evergreens and seven candles and processes through the house carrying a tray of coffee and Lucy buns to the bedroom of an adult member of the household (usually her mother) and followed by a retinue of handmaidens and star-boys, all singing Advent carols and songs. Saint Lucy's procession is also popular in hospitals and homes for the elderly.

Action

This Scandinavian custom could be easily adopted by any household with young children. It helps to focus the children's attention on the coming of the Divine Light into the world and very little is required in the way of 'props'. The procession does not have to take place at four in the morning! It happens at that time in Sweden only in order to avoid disrupting the working day, but it should, if possible, begin before daybreak.

Apart from the white dress and red ribbon or sash, you will need wands with a silver or gold star stuck on the top for the boys, a garland for the girl who is to be Saint Lucy and a tray of Lucy buns and coffee.

The crown can be made by fixing evergreens into the sort of metal base which is used for a bridesmaid's garland and is easily available at most florists. Holly is rather prickly, so it is best to stick to laurel and fir. Candles can be attached to the crown, using the sort of clips which are used for candles on Christmas trees, and a red ribbon is entwined in the leaves and tied at the back in a bow. In the interest of safety substitute artificial candles for the real ones particularly if the children are not going to be supervised.

Here is a traditional recipe for the Lucy buns:

INGREDIENTS

(175g (6oz) strong white bread-making flour (warmed, i.e. not out of a cold storage place)
(100/125g) 4oz butter or margarine
$\frac{1}{2}$ tsp salt
1 pinch saffron or 1 tsp ground cardamon
$\frac{1}{2}$ tsp sugar
1 pkt dried yeast
1 egg
142ml ($\frac{1}{4}$ pt) milk

Melt the butter or margarine in a saucepan. When it is melted, turn off the heat and add the milk, which should be just above blood temperature. Put half the amount of flour into a big bowl with the salt and dried yeast. Mix. Make a well in the flour mixture and pour in the warm or tepid milk and butter or margarine. Mix this well with a wooden spoon, gradually beating in the flour. If the mixture proves difficult to handle, turn it on to a floured surface and knead in any remaining flour. The dough should be soft and pliable.

Roll the dough into 15cm (6in) sausage lengths about the

thickness of a finger. Curl the ends of each length towards one another to form a crescent shape and place the crescents back to back on a greased baking sheet with a sultana in each corner for decoration. Leave them to rise for up to $1\frac{1}{2}$ hours, depending on the temperature of the room. Brush with milk and egg. Place on the top shelf of a fairly hot oven (200C, 400F, gas 6) for about 30 minutes.

Here are two additional ways of handling the dough:

1 Roll out to a flat strip. Spread evenly with butter or margarine. Sprinkle with cinnamon, sugar and dried fruit. Roll into a swiss roll. Cut these into $\frac{1}{2}$in pieces. Leave to rise and bake as above.
2 Treat as above (1) but instead of cutting the roll into pieces bake it in one in the middle of the oven (190C, 375F, gas 5).
   Turn the finished rolls on to a baking rack, covering them with towels to prevent them from becoming hard and crusty.

Third Sunday in Advent

Reading

Give ear, Lord, to our prayers and by thy gracious visitation lighten the darkness of our minds; through Jesus Christ, who lives and reigns with thee and the Holy Spirit, now and ever. Amen.

Collect

Meditation

Advent is, above all, a time of creative preparation, when we prepare ourselves inwardly and outwardly for the coming of the Saviour as the least and most insignificant among us. At the same time, we become aware of his promised return when we shall least expect him. The unpredictability of God is something to be wondered at continually.

Use this time to revisit in your own heart the manner of his gracious visitation. Had he chosen to be born in a palace, he would have been inaccessible to the vast majority of people and would remain so today. He comes in simplicity to prevent us from making of him an untouchable golden idol. He insists on being involved in our predicament, that we might reach out and touch him wherever we happen to be placed in life. He does not ask that we cry out our need for him with a loud voice because of his being in a far-off place, or one from which we are excluded. But he comes close to us, so that we may whisper to him our most secret fears and longings and so that he in turn may whisper comfort to hearts grown cold, and lighten the spiritual darkness of the modern mind.

Take the world you experience into the light of Christ and bring before him those known to you who live in the darkness of depression or fear. Bring especially those who believe that there is no hope for the future, no possibility for reconciliation or for a new beginning in countries which are torn apart by war. If you feel like this yourself, try to set aside, even if it is only for a moment, any tendency you may have to expect the worst from people and situations. Be fully present to hope. The acceptance in ourselves of the possible reconciliation in the world makes us ambassadors for Christ and messengers of hope. Hope, like despair, is contagious.

Action

Engage in creative action for the coming year. Contact someone you may be working with and establish lines of human contact. Suggest a coffee or a meal.

Saint Thomas the Apostle
21 December

Reading

Now Thomas, one of the twelve, called the Twin, was not with them when Jesus came. So the other disciples told him, 'We have seen the Lord.' But he said to them, 'Unless I see in his hands the print of the nails, and place my finger in the mark of the nails, and place my hand in his side, I will not believe.'

Eight days later, his disciples were again in the house, and Thomas was with them. The doors were shut, but Jesus came and stood among them, and said, 'Peace be with you.' Then he said to Thomas, 'Put your finger here, and see my hands; and put out your hand, and place it in my side; do not be faithless, but believing.' Thomas answered him, 'My Lord and my God!' Jesus said to him, 'Have you believed because you have seen me? Blessed are those who have not seen and yet believe' (John 20:24–30).

Meditation

The true meaning of the word 'blessed' is 'happy', so when we believe in God without seeing him we should count ourselves as happy. But faith is more than belief and the truly happy person, the person who is complete and whole, is the one who not only believes God and trusts him, but experiences God in his or her life. Faith makes it possible to let go of cosy beliefs so that we can apprehend with the eye of understanding the reality of God at work in our lives and in the world, even in the most desperate and apparently hopeless situations.

The myth of Father Christmas has its place in the order of things, in that to some extent, like all myths, it provides a brief escape from the mundane and the pragmatic, but it does not give us an abiding experience of Truth. Myths are like sweet fizzy drinks which provide only a temporary respite from thirst. The thirst very soon returns because only water can quench it. Similarly, only Christ can quench the very real thirst which we in the world have for a living truth in our lives.

The world reflects the state of our hearts which are inwardly lonely and much in need of his presence. To believe is not enough, but it is a beginning. We build on our believing and discover the reality of the risen Christ who has already united himself to us.

Action

If possible, spend some time with a child, preferably aged about three or four. Try to get on the same wavelength. Try to let go of adult common sense and 'believe' in the way the child believes. Talk without talking down to that child. Give your full attention and apprehend God and the world, if only for a brief moment, through the child's eyes. If your companion proves unco-operative, try again later in the week!

Fourth Sunday in Advent

Reading

Rejoice in the Lord always; again I will say, rejoice. Let your gentleness be known to everyone. The Lord is near. Do not worry about anything, but in everything by prayer and supplication with thanksgiving let your requests be made known to God. And the peace of God, which surpasses all understanding, will guard your hearts and your minds in Christ Jesus.

Finally, beloved, whatever is true, whatever is honourable, whatever is just, whatever is pure, whatever is pleasing, whatever is commendable, if there is any excellence and if there is anything worthy of praise, think about these things. Keep on doing the things that you have learned and received and heard and seen in me, and the God of peace will be with you (Phil. 4:4–9 NRSV).

Meditation

Bright smiles do not necessarily convey joy, for Christian joy is far more than superficial optimism. It is won through suffering. It comes of an intimate knowledge, a first-hand experience of Christ in our darkest moments and in the ability to allow him into the darkest recesses of our personality. It comes of the acceptance of his presence within ourselves, our society and the created world around us. Christian joy comes out of detecting the imprint of his features in those of our neighbour and in the transcendent beauty of the natural world. His features being so deeply engraved in our own hearts should make us attracted to the people and things which enable us to focus on the living presence of Christ in our midst.

Action

Avoid for today amusements or activities which distract the heart from Christ. Instead, set aside a little time to think on what is gracious and worthy of praise. Drop into an art gallery or museum. Go to a concert. Read a poem. Do any or all of these things with a heart open to receiving the experience of the living God.

CHRISTMASTIDE

Christmas Eve

Reading

I am the Alpha and the Omega (Rev. 21:6).

Meditation

The beginning and the end, the source and the life, come in quietness and poverty to meet us in the silence of our hearts and in the poverty of our human state. The great Lord of Creation comes to us out of the silence that gave meaning and form to the word 'existence'. He leaves behind the power and the glory of heaven and comes silently to those who will receive him in simplicity and love. The Lord of Creation is simply and silently in our midst and invites us to meet him by 'being' in him in simplicity.

We drop into that place of inner silence which is the home God has chosen for himself, our own individual Bethlehem. A heart which is indwelt by Christ in this way is a place of refuge from the glitz, greed and noise of a commercial Christmas. It is the inner sanctuary where a person experiences God, for Christ did not come merely to fulfil prophecy, or to bequeath to us a code of conduct with the hope of heaven at some time in the future, but that we might experience him fully and continually for ourselves.

Action

Keep aside a moment today, even if it is only a single minute in the busy day full of last-minute preparations, for encountering the Christ-child in your own deep inner silence. Let a simple task or action affirm this moment of encounter, when face to face you meet him and feel the warmth of his smile. The wrapping of a present, or the preparation of a stocking for a particular individual can serve as a way of consecrating, in the silence of the heart, all the giving and the celebrating that are to take place in the coming week.

Christmas Day

Reading

For to us a child is born, to us a son is given (Isa. 9:6).

Meditation

In all the excitement of giving and receiving; of presents, of food that has been prepared in the past weeks, of having with us friends and relatives whom we do not see all the time, we are inwardly glad and thankful for the gift of our humanity and for the gift of life in all its forms.

Christ comes to be one with us in our human predicament. He visits us silently in our secret heart and comes unnoticed, in the stranger or in a person whom we take for granted. The world smothers him in tinsel or in the noise and vapid imagery of a commercial Christmas, but we cleave inwardly to the sure knowledge that God so loves us that he desires to be an integral part of our human experience, so that even in moments which are stressful and full of discord, we hold the Christ-child in the intimacy of our hearts and are thankful that he has been given to us.

Action

In opening a present, or in thanking someone for something which is much appreciated, or if a quarrel breaks out, make room in your heart, in the safe place of your inner silence, for the Christ-child and thank God for the gift of himself.

Saint Stephen
26 December

Reading

Good King Wenceslas look'd out
On the feast of Stephen,
When the snow lay round about
Deep and crisp and even:
Brightly shone the moon that night,
Though the frost was cruel,
When a poor man came in sight,
Gath'ring winter fuel.

'Hither, page, and stand by me,
If thou know'st it, telling,
Yonder peasant, who is he?
Where and what his dwelling?'
'Sire, he lives a good league hence,
Underneath the mountain,
Right against the forest fence,
By Saint Agnes' fountain.'

'Bring me flesh and bring me wine,
Bring me pine-logs hither:
Thou and I will see him dine,
When we bear them thither.'
Page and monarch, forth they went,
Forth they went together;
Through the rude wind's wild lament
And the bitter weather.

'Sire, the night is darker now,
And the wind blows stronger;
Fails my heart, I know not how;
I can go no longer.'
'Mark my foot-steps, good my page;
Tread thou in them boldly:
Thou shalt find the winter's rage
Freeze thy blood less coldly.'

In his master's steps he trod,
Where the snow lay dinted;
Heat was in the very sod
Which the saint had printed.
Therefore, Christian men be sure,
Wealth or rank possessing,
Ye who now will bless the poor,
Shall yourselves find blessing.

Meditation

Saint Stephen, the first Christian martyr, was also the first
deacon. The Greek word for deacon is *diakonos*, meaning
servant. Good King Wenceslas is really a Christ figure, and his
relationship with his servant illustrates the Christian's relationship with Christ our master. But Stephen is also a Christ
figure, for Christ himself becomes our servant, so when we
pattern our lives on his by patterning them in love on his
example, we find that the lack of love in the world – 'the
winter's rage' – freezes our blood less coldly.

We serve Christ in serving those around us, from our
immediate neighbours and those with whom we live, to the
oppressed and the poor of the earth. Service can take the form
of action, or of simply opening one's heart in compassion to a
person's or a nation's suffering. We serve others in recognising
them as unique individuals by affirming the Christ in them.

Our attitude to other people, whether they are close friends or strangers, is a good indicator of the extent to which we are capable of allowing them a share in our personal experience of Christ's love.

Action

Today is also Boxing Day when traditionally tradespeople were given 'boxes' containing some sort of gratuity, so set aside a small gift ready for whoever delivers your milk or post, or collects your rubbish. Hand it to them personally, along with a greeting or a smile which comes from a real desire for their well-being and happiness.

Hanukkah
Jewish Feast of Rededication

Reading

Blessed art thou O Lord our God who has sanctified us by thy commandments and has commanded us to kindle the light of Hanukkah . . . Blessed art thou O Lord our God who achieved miracles for our forefathers in days of old at this season . . . O fortress, rock of my salvation unto thee it is becoming to give praise.

Prayers and blessings recited during
the season of Hanukkah

Meditation

Christianity has its roots in Judaism. The Jews are our direct spiritual ancestors, so we enrich our spiritual lives by linking up with the Jewish feasts which fall at a similar time to our own.

Hanukkah, like Christmas, coincides with the darkest time of the year. A candle is lit each night for eight successive nights, to correspond with the gradual lengthening of days after the winter solstice.

The feast was established in thanksgiving for the deliverance of the Jewish people from the oppression of the Greek emperor Antiochus who not only profaned Jewish temples and tried to expunge Jewish culture and language from the face of the earth, but even conferred upon himself the title of 'Theos epiphanes' or 'God made manifest'. He was ultimately defeated by Judas Maccabeus in the rebellion of 165 BC when the temple was recaptured, cleansed and rededicated.

The Jewish people light candles to remember when they

were delivered from persecution and darkness. We light
candles in our churches in honour of Christ, the light of
the world, who delivers us from the darkness of an existence
without God. So take time today, perhaps when lighting a
candle, to hold in your heart a world which for the most part
turns its back on God and on the immensity of his love.

Own before God whatever feelings emerge, allowing at the
same time whatever person or group of people who surface in
your heart to be especially loved by God at this particular
moment. Don't work at this by trying frantically to remember
all the people and situations who need your prayers while you
seem to have all the right feelings. Stay with whoever comes to
mind, whatever the feelings, and if compassion for them
should return unexpectedly at some point in the day, stay
with it for as long as you can. It is important to remember that
we are never alone when we pray, especially when we pray for
others and that we do nothing in our own strength but only in
what is given to us by the Spirit of God.

Action

You can read about the Maccabean Revolt in the Book of
Maccabees in the Apocryphal section of the Bible.

Here is a recipe for potato *latkes* which are traditionally eaten
at this time:

INGREDIENTS

6 medium sized potatoes
1 small onion (optional)
2 eggs slightly beaten
3 tbsp flour
$\frac{1}{4}$ tsp pepper
1 tsp salt
$\frac{1}{2}$ tsp baking powder

Peel and grate the potatoes and onion. Allow them to stand for 10 minutes so that the liquid rises to the top. Remove the liquid and stir in the eggs. Add the other ingredients. Drop by spoonsful on to a hot, well-greased skillet. Drain on absorbent paper. Serve hot with apple sauce, sugar, or sour cream.

The Holy Innocents
28 December

Reading

Now when they had departed, behold, an angel of the Lord appeared to Joseph in a dream and said, 'Rise, take the child and his mother, and flee to Egypt, and remain there till I tell you; for Herod is about to search for the child, to destroy him.' And he rose and took the child and his mother by night, and departed to Egypt and remained there until the death of Herod.

Then Herod, when he saw that he had been tricked by the wise men, was in a furious rage, and he sent and killed all the male children in Bethlehem and all that region who were two years old or under, according to the time which he had ascertained from the wise men (Matt. 2:13–15, 16).

Meditation

These small children are the first in a long line of innocent victims who have been persecuted and killed for Christ's sake. We do not understand why suffering is allowed. Many people find it incompatible with the idea of a loving and all-powerful God. But Christ comes to join in with our situation, so that in suffering we are united to him.

We place ourselves mentally in the position of Joseph who carries such responsibility and we identify with his fears and doubts. We experience with Mary the fear of exile and of the idea of travelling with a young child in such difficult and dangerous circumstances.

According to one legend, on the first night of their journey the Holy Family found a cave to shelter in. A spider, who normally inhabited the cave, recognised the Christ-child and wanted to make him a gift. His only talent was that of weaving webs, so to please the child and to shelter him from the bitter night wind, he decided to weave a huge and intricate web across the entrance to the cave. In the morning, drops of dew settled on the web, and when a company of Roman soldiers came searching for the child in order to kill him, they noticed the web and assuming, quite logically, that it had been there for some time, passed on without bothering to search the cave.

Action

If by any chance you know of a child who is teased at school, seek out him or her and offer sympathy and help. Encourage other children to give their support.

I have always felt differently about spiders since I heard this story, so perhaps it would be worth reappraising our attitudes to these creatures.

Christmas Octave

Reading

*Grant, we pray thee, almighty God, that thy only-begotten Son's
new birth as man may deliver us, whom the old slavery holds fast
beneath the yoke of sin.*

Collect for the Christmas Octave

Meditation

The wooden yoke of service to self, to the 'I' becomes the
wood of the cross, the vertical beam which carries the weight
of the Saviour. It becomes the wood of the manger in which
the Christ-child is laid in poverty and humility and the wood
which was chiselled and sawed by the hands of the carpenter's
apprentice in the workshop in Nazareth.

God comes in human form to deliver us from slavery to the
self; in other words to the ego, in order that we might have our
true self returned to us, re-created and freed into his image and
likeness. We were fashioned in the image of God. This is not
an image which is ready made and separate from us, like a
picture or statue, but one which is repeated in a million diverse
ways throughout our physical makeup and psyche. We are
made through and through like the God who loves us, but we
are also free to mar that image and to create for ourselves
other gods, limited to the confines of our human desires and of
our limited understanding.

'The yoke of sin' comes from the inability to understand
what it means to be fully human and yet made in the image

and likeness of God. Such understanding comes with a wholehearted desire to know God, not from intellectual curiosity (although that is important) but from a love which is born from the recognition of a fundamental need both in the individual and in society. Desire and love for God must not be limited to 'me and my personal salvation' but must embrace the anguish and loneliness of the world.

Action

Be disposed to do someone a favour, even if it disrupts your plans.

The Naming of Jesus
1 January

Reading

*Almighty God, who has given thy Son Jesus Christ the Name
which is above every name, and has taught us that there is none
other whereby we may be saved: grant that rejoicing in his Name
we may ever strive to proclaim it to all people; through the same
Jesus Christ our Lord. Amen.*

Collect

Meditation

The fact that God consents to be named at all is in itself an
unfathomable mystery. In biblical times, his chosen people
worshipped him from afar. He hid himself in a pillar of flame
and in a great cloud. Even the mountain on which he was
manifested to Moses was forbidden to both humans and
animals, on pain of death by stoning. God was unapproachable and unnameable. He was Yahweh, Jehovah, Eloim –
names which attempted to convey, and at the same time
conceal from crude human understanding, the mysterious,
multifaceted, inexpressible nature of the Godhead, a Godhead
whose persona lay beyond the confines of gender, and yet was
complete and whole as both masculine and feminine.

The unapproachable and unnameable God of Abraham
and Moses draws near to us in the person and name of Jesus, a
name which means 'Jehovah is salvation'. The saving nature
of God is affirmed in the man Jesus who is the risen Christ. His
power to heal and make whole remains undiminished, as it

was in the time of Moses and during his earthly ministry, and as it will continue to be to the end of the last age.

Action

Now is the time for New Year resolutions. Let this year begin and end with reverence and love for the Lord's name. When the name of Jesus is invoked as a swear word, or taken lightly, the Orthodox Jesus Prayer said from the heart is an excellent means of atonement: 'Lord Jesus Christ, Son of God, have mercy.'

Saint Macarius the Younger
2 January

Reading

I give glory to thee, O God, who wast with Daniel in the lion's den, who didst give understanding unto beasts.

Prayer of St Macarius of Alexandria

Meditation

A desert hermit of the fourth century, Macarius is particularly remembered for his great love of wild animals. On one occasion a hyena brought her blind whelp to the entrance of his cave and with a touch of the saint's hand the animal's sight was restored. The mother was said to have brought him a sheepskin as a token of her gratitude, but Macarius, out of his great love for all of God's creation, made her promise never to take life again and only to eat animals which were already dead. He guaranteed to feed her with bread on the days when she was unable to find food.

Macarius is also said to have been so smitten with shame at having swatted a mosquito that he betook himself to a swamp which was infested with these creatures and lived there for several months. Whether or not we view this sort of ascetic practice as excessive, it is still worth examining our own attitudes to animals and insects, for God is to be found and adored in all of life.

Look out of the nearest window and simply take in the sky, the cloud formations, the quality of the light. If it is dark wrap the protective cloak of night and of the silence of the small hours around your own heart and be given over to gratitude to God whose mysterious name is whispered to us in the wind and rain, in the distant bark of a dog and in all the animal life around us which we so often take for granted. Imagine for a moment what human existence would be like without the placid company of animals and be grateful for them.

Action

It may be true that the earth can only support a limited number of vegetarians, but we must nevertheless consume our meat with humility and gratitude, realising that we too are of flesh and blood, and will one day come to die. If you have a local butcher, make sure you know where and how the meat on offer is slaughtered and what sort of conditions the creatures have been living in prior to being killed. You can also write to your local supermarket expressing similar concerns.

EPIPHANYTIDE

The Epiphany of Our Lord
6 January

Reading

For the grace of God has appeared, bringing salvation to all, training us to renounce impiety and worldly passions, and in the present age to live lives that are self-controlled, upright, and godly, while we wait for the blessed hope and the manifestation of the glory of our great God and Saviour Jesus Christ. He it is who gave himself for us that he might redeem us from all iniquity and purify for himself a people of his own who are zealous for good deeds (Titus 2:11–14).

> Epistle for the Orthodox Liturgy on the Feast of The Holy Theophany of Our Lord And Saviour Jesus Christ.

Meditation

The word 'epiphany' comes from the Greek *epiphanes*, meaning 'to make manifest', so today we celebrate the revealing of the Christ-child to the whole world; not just to one group of people, be they Christians or Jews, but to all nations. In certain countries it is the day of present-giving, in memory of the wise men who visited the Child and his mother and brought him prophetic gifts of gold, frankincense and myrrh.

It is also a time for planning the year ahead, for plotting our course over the coming months, as the wise men plotted a course across the desert, guided by the new star. Today, we often overplan our lives, so that we miss out on the opportunities and joys of the present moment and leave very little to God who loves to surprise us with sudden and unexpected manifestations of his presence.

No matter how well we plan things, we still live with uncertainty, in a time of waiting – waiting for the inevitable end to our lives on earth and waiting as a human family for the coming of the Son of Man in great glory. When viewed in this way, waiting and uncertainty cease to be a matter of twiddling one's thumbs in the fond hope that life will all of a sudden be made easier. Times of uncertainty and waiting become opportunities for creative and active engagement in the business of making the world a better place by the extent to which we are able to manifest the love of the living God from our own hearts. We are dealing here with compassion, which has little to do with 'caring' and 'sharing', the empty catch-words which have become worn out through overuse.

In planning the year which lies ahead, allow for the fact that true compassion frequently makes unexpected demands on our time and can ruin the best laid plans.

Action

Be open to God's plan for the future and to his presence here and now. Get into the habit of combining projects and plans with the words, 'God willing' from the Latin *Deo volente*, usually shortened to DV. A similar phrase is used in the Islamic world, '*En ch'allah*'.

First Sunday in Epiphany

Reading

Yet now take courage, O Zerubbabel, says the Lord; take courage, O Joshua, son of Jehozadak, the high priest; take courage, all you people of the land, says the Lord; work, for I am with you says the Lord of hosts, according to the promise that I made you when you came out of Egypt. My Spirit abides among you; fear not. For thus says the Lord of hosts: Once again, in a little while, I will shake the heavens and the earth and the sea and the dry land; and I will shake all nations, so that the treasures of all nations shall come in, and I will fill this house with splendour, says the Lord of hosts. The silver is mine, and the gold is mine, says the Lord of hosts. The latter splendour of this house shall be greater than the former, says the Lord of hosts; and in this place I will give prosperity, says the Lord of hosts (Hag. 2:4–9).

Meditation

We live in exciting times. Throughout this century, right up to the present day, a great reordering has been taking place in the world. It has often involved much suffering, but it has also brought out courage and compassion on the part of individuals and of nations. Hitherto insurmountable barriers have been overturned and God has shown us that, even in modern times, he is still at work bringing his people out of captivity. For it is people who are the 'treasures of all nations': the indomitable spirit of human beings in their quest for political or personal freedom is no less than God's own Spirit abiding and working with them. We must look, therefore, with courage and with eager anticipation, to the days when the world, the Church and our inmost selves will be shaken down to reveal that which is truly of God.

We are to take courage, even when the world seems plunged in darkness. For God intervenes in his own time and shakes all nations, as he has done in the Communist world and in South Africa, and as he does in the heart and mind of the individual who seeks him in truth and sincerity. We are to take courage; so this week confront a fear, whether it has to do with the future, with yourself or with a relationship. Taking courage means just that; taking hold of the courage which is our gift from God's Holy Spirit, and looking fear in the eye, by first admitting it to ourselves and then by allowing God to take hold of the fear for us, that he might be made manifest even at the heart of a private terror.

Action

Own your most secret fear, no matter how silly or unimportant it may seem. Do so, knowing that there is not a person on earth who is not afraid of something, for we are all deficient in love, and it is only perfect love which casts out fear. Forgive yourself for this deficiency and for being afraid. Try to bring that secret fear out into the open and ask for God's help to tackle it firmly and overcome it.

The Baptism of Our Lord

Reading

Behold the Lamb of God, who takes away the sin of the world (John 1:29).

Meditation

We place ourselves alongside those who have come to be baptised in the Jordan and try to experience, rather than merely understand intellectually, the feelings which John the Baptist experiences on seeing Jesus walking towards him. The whole point of his ministry is revealed in this moment. The prophecy is fulfilled, the faith and courage of a lifetime of witnessing under threat of persecution are rewarded. We experience with John, as we meet the eyes of Christ, the one who takes away what might also be termed the grief of the world. For sin is not mere wrongdoing, but an occasion for grief, as it is the trampling and soiling of God's image in the world and in ourselves. We know from the heart the wonder of Christ's baptism which affirms our kinship with him.

Action

It is important to let this kind of meditation, in which we place ourselves in the context of an event in the life of Christ, take its own course. It is very much a matter of allowing things to happen in the way in which God chooses, so the action, if there is to be an action, will be made quite clear during the course of the prayer. However, what can be very helpful is the keeping of a journal or prayer diary in which we jot down the things which came through most clearly in the meditation, so that we can return to them later and understand them at a deeper level. There is no need to write reams. A few sentences or points will be enough.

Saint Anthony of Egypt
17 January

Reading

Blessed are those who trust in the Lord, whose trust is the Lord. They shall be like a tree planted by water, sending out its roots by the stream. It shall not fear when heat comes, for its leaves shall stay green; in the year of drought it is not anxious, and it does not cease to bear fruit (Jer. 17: 7–8 NRSV).

Meditation

Saint Anthony is best remembered for the great agony of mind which he endured in the desert. His desert was metaphorical, as well as physical, for there is no greater loneliness than battling with temptation, no matter how mundane the temptation may be. His call to the life of a hermit came to him one day when he heard the words, 'If thou wilt be perfect, go, sell what thou hast and give to the poor; and come and follow me, and thou shalt have treasure in heaven.'

We are all called to have this attitude to our possessions if we are truly to think of ourselves as disciples of Christ. But poverty is not an end in itself. It is the means to true wealth and freedom. Freedom from an excess of material wealth brings eventually a surprising freedom from the desire for it. When the gifts which the world has to bestow are seen for what they really are, and cease to matter all that much, we realise increasingly the true value of the gifts which come from God. In today's world they amount to freedom from anxiety (less stress) and freedom from desire (less time wasted in pursuing the things which disrupt relationships and which in themselves do not make for happiness).

Anthony's holiness was a gift bestowed on him by God, who taught him through adversity that his true wealth lay in having Christ with him at all times, even in periods of darkness. Trust is not just a matter of believing that God is vaguely around, but of actively going forward to meet him and in so doing, being prepared to leave everything else behind. By clinging less and less to material things and personal attributes, we shall not cease to bear fruit. On the contrary, we shall become like a tree which grows imperceptibly and without effort.

Action

If practical, plant a tree or a rose, bearing in mind as you do how the young plant will flourish over the years, given the right conditions, and how its growth will not depend on its striving or being anxious about the next rainfall. It will simply get on with the business of growing, and so give glory to God. If tree-planting is not an option, try starting a few seedlings in a seed tray, or even some mustard and cress on a piece of blotting paper.

Second Sunday in Epiphany

Reading

Thus says God, the Lord, who created the heavens and stretched them out, who spread forth the earth and what comes from it, who gives breath to the people upon it and spirit to those who walk in it: 'I am the Lord, I have called you in righteousness, I have taken you by the hand and kept you; I have given you as a covenant to the people, a light to the nations, to open the eyes that are blind, to bring out the prisoners from the dungeon, from the prison those who sit in darkness' (Isa. 42:5–7).

Meditation

The full purpose of the Passion is triumphantly consummated in the Resurrection, but it begins in secret in the Incarnation and is first revealed in the Epiphany, the manifestation of Christ to a benighted world.

Even today, Christ continues to be a living reality, a miracle of light in the darkness of our daily tribulations, when for a moment we sense that something greater than our own pain and our own individuality lies beyond what we experience.

Pain and suffering do not usually disappear with prayer which, rather than being a shopping list of requests, ought to be an act of surrender, of joining ourselves to God, heart to heart. Because of our union with God, we are not alone in pain. Christ, the light of the world, has arrived there before us and meets us in adversity, so that we, in whom the light of Christ shines, may be a light to others.

Action

Be open and completely present to the pain of another person, beginning with a member of your own household whose pain you may think you already know. Charity really does begin at home. Try, even though it may be painful, really to experience their predicament and what causes them to be who they are and what they are. Understanding a person means forgetting oneself completely for a time and getting into their skin, as it were. Christ who is the light in our darkness seeks to do this in us all the time and asks that we do the same for one another.

Third Sunday in Epiphany

Reading

Now the boy Samuel was ministering to the Lord under Eli. And the word of the Lord was rare in those days; there was no frequent vision.

At that time Eli, whose eyesight had begun to grow dim, so that he could not see, was lying down in his own place; the lamp of God had not yet gone out, and Samuel was lying down within the temple of the Lord, where the ark of God was. Then the Lord called, 'Samuel! Samuel!' and he said, 'Here I am!' and ran to Eli, and said, 'Here I am, for you called me.' But he said, 'I did not call; lie down again.' So he went and lay down. And the Lord called again, 'Samuel!' And Samuel arose and went to Eli, and said, 'Here I am, for you called me.' But he said, 'I did not call, my son; lie down again.' Now Samuel did not yet know the Lord, and the word of the Lord had not yet been revealed to him. And the Lord called Samuel again the third time. And he arose and went to Eli, and said, 'Here I am, for you called me.' Then Eli perceived that the Lord was calling the boy. Therefore Eli said to Samuel, 'Go, lie down; and if he calls you, you shall say, "Speak, Lord, for thy servant hears."' So Samuel went and lay down in his place (1 Sam. 3:1–9).

Meditation

Samuel 'did not yet know the Lord'. He received the call of God into a heart which was not only pure (his youthful innocence seems to shine through this passage) but which was as yet untouched by the hand of God. When we are touched by God, when we experience him, life is never quite the same again. Experiencing God in the way Samuel experienced him is a great privilege, not something to feel pious or smug about. It requires that we be ready and available at all times and in all places for God to manifest himself to us and as a result of this, be prepared to be totally given over to the service of others.

In Samuel's day the word of the Lord and frequent visions were rare, as they are today, because of the spiritual deafness which prevailed in that society, as it does in our own. 'Visions' and 'voices' are not necessary in order to hear and experience God's Holy Spirit. In fact, these phenomena are on the whole best suited to the very young who can take such things in their stride, or to people with nerves of steel. What is needful, however, is a pure heart, like that of Samuel and his master Eli, well tuned to the voice of God speaking in the heart, in other words to the reality of the kingdom of heaven within us. This should be the attribute of every Christian.

Action

Make a list of the things which claim your attention. Are they truly productive and life enhancing? Do they leave a space for God's voice?

Saint Thomas Aquinas
28 January

Reading

God's spirit is said to move over the waters as an artist's will moves over the material to be shaped by his art.

From *Summa Theologica*

Meditation

The platonic idea of God was that he was the 'unmoved mover'. All life had its origin in this nebulous entity which depended on nothing for its existence. For us, God is the one through whom all things were made 'and without him was not anything made that was made'. He exists outside time and space and has his beginning in a time before the beginning of time, as the Word (or in French *le verbe* which implies action and motivation) and 'from his fullness have we all received grace upon grace'.

Our free will is an inalienable gift, given to us by God that we might share with him as artists of life and stewards of the universe in the process of creation. In this respect, human beings occupy a more privileged position in the heavenly hierarchy than the mightiest angel, for in every person on earth exists the potential for divinisation, for being like Christ.

Our lives and all the possibilities open to us are the raw material with which as artists we fashion our own destiny, choosing in every second, between the great master plan of the Creator and our own short-sighted perception of what we need in order to be happy. Our individual lives and the destiny of the whole human race are inextricably linked. They are part of the great canvas on which we are privileged to work alongside the Master and which we shall one day see completed.

Action

Take some clay and allow it to take form in your hands. All creativity is a process of standing back and allowing. Paint a picture. Decorate a wall. Any action which is aimed at bringing into existence something that hitherto did not exist focuses the heart and mind on our co-creatorship with God.

The Presentation of Christ
in the Temple
Candlemas, 2 February

Reading

Lord, now lettest thou thy servant depart in peace, according to thy word; for mine eyes have seen thy salvation which thou hast prepared in the presence of all peoples, a light for revelation to the Gentiles, and for glory to thy people Israel (Luke 2:29–32).

Meditation

Christ is to be our glory, as we are his glory. We are called to reflect the light of Christ by living fully in him as the human beings which we were created to be. In this way, others will recognise him in us, as Simeon recognised him from among the many small babies whom he must have held in his arms at the time of their presentation.

This is a good opportunity to change places with Simeon and Anna and to experience from the heart, without straining with the intellect, what it is to hold the Christ-child, to feel his human weight and to look into his eyes. Try to experience in this moment the utter dependence of Christ on the individuals and on the society to which he chose to belong and how, from the very beginning, he puts himself at our mercy. '*Kyrie Eleison*' – 'Lord have mercy', is a heartfelt response to the wonder of God's humility in making himself so vulnerable to us.

Action

Traditionally, Candlemas was the feast on which the Church blessed all the candles to be used in ceremonies throughout the year. It was a custom designed to celebrate Christ as 'a light for revelation to the Gentiles, and for glory to thy people Israel'.

Here is a recipe for floating candles, the simplest way to make candles at home:

You will need:

  4 large walnuts
  12in (32cm) narrow candle wicking
  Paraffin wax
  Impact adhesive
  Sharp handicraft knife
  Cooking thermometer

To make:

Using the knife, carefully halve the walnuts and remove the contents of each shell. Heat the wax to 82°C (180°F). Cut the wicking into eight 1½in (4cm) lengths. Knot one end of each length, then dip in wax and pull straight. Place a blob of impact adhesive centrally in the base of each nutshell and push the knotted end of the wicks on top, with the help of a matchstick, so that the wicks stand up vertically. Stand the shells in an old egg box and leave the glue to dry. Fill the shells with wax. Allow it to set, then top up round the wick. Float the walnut shells in a shallow dish of water.

Fourth Sunday in Epiphany

Reading

On the third day there was a marriage at Cana in Galilee, and the mother of Jesus was there; Jesus also was invited to the marriage, with his disciples. When the wine gave out, the mother of Jesus said to him, 'They have no wine.' And Jesus said to her, 'O woman, what have you to do with me? My hour has not yet come.' His mother said to the servants, 'Do whatever he tells you.' Now six stone jars were standing there, for the Jewish rites of purification, each holding twenty or thirty gallons. Jesus said to them, 'Fill the jars with water.' And they filled them up to the brim. He said to them, 'Now draw some out, and take it to the steward of the feast.' So they took it. When the steward of the feast tasted the water now become wine, and did not know where it came from (though the servants who had drawn the water knew), the steward of the feast called the bridegroom and said to him, 'Every man serves the good wine first; and when men have drunk freely, then the poor wine; but you have kept the good wine until now.' This, the first of his signs, Jesus did at Cana in Galilee, and manifested his glory; and his disciples believed in him. (John 2:1–11).

Meditation

It is significant that the first miracle which Jesus performed, even before his hour had come, was to save a party from disaster. No situation is too insignificant for the Saviour of the world to enter into and buy back. This is his first recorded act of saving, of restoring and making whole a situation which was in danger of being broken and damaged, for the guests would all go home if the wine ran out, and the young couple would be left with an embarrassing and miserable end to their wedding celebrations.

Be present at this party as a wedding guest, a parent of the bride or groom, or as one of the two getting married. Be aware of the full implicatios of their dilemma, perhaps by placing the situation in a modern context – a reception which for some reason has gone badly wrong. Seek out the Lord in the crowd, or his mother, or one of his friends. Give yourself enough time to experience fully whatever feelings come as a result of what he says to you. If you decide to follow up with the action on the next page, let the supper party you are preparing be a symbol of the party of life itself and a reminder of the Eucharist and the heavenly banquet which we have been promised in the next life.

Christ came into the world to celebrate life with us and to consecrate and draw us to himself in all circumstances.

Action

Give a party or invite a few friends for supper. Be truly glad and grateful for fun and fellowship, and for everything that celebrates life.

CHICKEN BAMIA

Here is a dish made with chicken and okra which can be made in advance and works equally well for a large number of people as for a small supper party. It is a recipe which originates in Iraq, but which is also popular among Palestinians.

INGREDIENTS FOR 6

1½lb fresh okra
(tinned will do, but will need less cooking time)
5 tbsp olive oil
2 thinly sliced onions
2 crushed cloves of garlic
1lb tomatoes, peeled and sliced or a 14oz tin
1 tsp each of turmeric, coriander, salt and freshly ground
   cumin
½ tsp black pepper
6 chicken pieces
Juice and rind of 1 lemon

A couple of hours before beginning to cook, dry the chicken pieces with a paper towel and rub them with a couple of pinches of salt and a pinch or two of turmeric for each piece. Leave to stand.

If using fresh okra wash them thoroughly and cut off the stems. Heat the oil in a large heavy-bottomed frying pan or pot and sauté the chicken pieces in it until lightly browned. Remove to a warm place. Now sauté the onions and garlic until they are soft. Add the remaining spices and the okra. Stir gently for a minute or two. Add the tomatoes, salt and pepper, followed by the chicken. If you are using fresh tomatoes you will need to add enough water at this stage to cover the chicken pieces. Tinned tomatoes are more liquid, so will need less water. Add the lemon juice and, if you want a more lemony flavour, the two halves of the lemon. Simmer for 45 minutes to an hour, or until the chicken is tender. If you have an Aga or Rayburn the dish will cook quite happily in the oven.

Serve with rice and a green salad with a bottle of red wine and some pitta bread to mop up the juice.

Fifth Sunday in Epiphany

Reading

For thus said the Lord God, the Holy One of Israel, 'In returning and rest you shall be saved; in quietness and in trust shall be your strength.' And you would not, but you said, 'No! We will speed upon horses,' therefore you shall speed away; and, 'We will ride upon swift steeds,' therefore your pursuers shall be swift. A thousand shall flee at the threat of one, at the threat of five you shall flee, till you are left like a flagstaff on the top of a mountain, like a signal on a hill. Therefore the Lord waits to be gracious to you; therefore he exalts himself to show mercy to you. For the Lord is a God of justice; blessed are all those who wait for him (Isa. 30:15–18).

Meditation

'In returning and rest you shall be saved;' The Greek word for repentance is *'metanoia'* which means to reorientate oneself, to return or to go back on one's tracks. Repentance should be thought of as an occasion for rejoicing and for rest, rather than as a depressing and somewhat self-indulgent 'guilt trip'. It is a time of shedding burdens, like taking off a coat on a warm day or of finding the right direction after much time spent getting more and more off course. The burden which we shed, the coat which we take off, is all the hurt we have experienced in our life. Once this coat has been shed we are better able to see the hurt we have inflicted on others in our preoccupation with our 'selves'. This preoccupation is very often manifested in our fundamental attitude towards God.

Nothing fits or works in life if God is not at the centre of it. In the rushing and grasping of modern life we 'speed upon horses', pursuing selfish or futile ends only to find ourselves alone 'like a flagstaff on the top of a mountain'. It is therefore important to take time for rest, in order that we may be able to reassess our aims and values, and to ask God for the grace and the courage to shed those attitudes and priorities which prevent us from hearing the voice of the one who guides us in the way each of us must walk, knowing that his growing presence in our lives is itself our true reward.

Action

Take time today to waste time. Spend ten minutes or so doing nothing in particular. If you find yourself idly staring out of a window or engaged in something which brings you peace but which is not necessarily 'productive', allow it to be, enjoy it. Have that second cup of coffee, or spend ten more minutes in bed or in the bath. God often speaks most clearly in such moments.

Septuagesima Sunday
Ninth before Easter

Reading

Now there is in Jerusalem by the Sheep Gate a pool, in Hebrew called Beth-zatha, which has five porticoes. In these lay a multitude of invalids, blind, lame, paralysed. One man was there, who had been ill for thirty-eight years. When Jesus saw him and knew that he had been lying there a long time, he said to him, 'Do you want to be healed?' The sick man answered him, 'Sir, I have no one to put me into the pool when the water is troubled, and while I am going another steps down before me.' Jesus said to him, 'Rise, take up your pallet, and walk.' And at once the man was healed, and he took up his pallet and walked (John 5:2–9).

Meditation

Disease, in the time of Christ, was often taken to be a punishment for sin. Although Jesus makes it quite clear on another occasion (see John 9:1–3) that this is not the case, he does use instances of disease to point to our need for inner healing and wholeness. Disease is a word whose root meaning is that all is not 'at ease' in us and the crucial question which is put to the man by the pool, 'Do you *want* to be healed?' is also put to us in connection with the healing of our own inner hurts and grievances, as well as with the healing of our physical diseases. This is not to say that physical illness is 'all in the mind' but many people unconsciously prolong illness because they so badly need the extra love which physical infirmity can attract. Doctors and nurses, as well as parents and anyone who cares for a sick person, are direct agents and transmitters of the love of God, whether they know it or not. Physical disease is not a punishment for sin but part of the Fall itself, a sin against creation.

Spiritual infirmity, like physical disease, is a missing of the mark and a falling short of the ideal. Spiritual sickness, no matter what form it takes (depression, in one form or another, is its most common manifestation) blocks love, and in so doing prevents people from becoming fully themselves, as they were created to be. By the very fact that we are so accustomed to them, our spiritual infirmities (our sins) can themselves become a crutch which prevents us from walking upright as complete human beings.

Experience what it feels like to be the man who has been paralysed for a very long time and look into the eyes of Christ as he asks, 'Do you want to be healed?'

Action

If you know someone suffering from the sort of illness which could be alleviated by a change in their own attitudes (such as eating disorders) spend some time with them with a view to achieving this.

Sexagesima Sunday
Eighth before Easter

Reading

You were dead through the trespasses and sins in which you once lived, following the course of this world, following the ruler of the power of the air, the spirit that is now at work among those who are disobedient. All of us once lived among them in the passions of our flesh, following the desires of flesh and senses and we were by nature children of wrath, like everyone else. But God, who is rich in mercy, out of the great love with which he loved us, even when we were dead through our trespasses, made us alive together with Christ – by grace you have been saved – and raised us up with him, and seated us with him in the heavenly places in Christ Jesus, so that in the ages to come he might show the immeasurable riches of his grace in kindness toward us in Christ Jesus. For by grace you have been saved through faith, and this is not your own doing; it is the gift of God – not the result of works, so that no one may boast. For we are what he has made us, created in Christ Jesus for good works, which God prepared beforehand to be our way of life (Eph. 2:1–10 NRSV).

Meditation

The absence of God's Holy Spirit continually remaking us from within reduces life to mere existence. Once, when I was on the top deck of a London bus which was slowly making its way down Oxford Street, I was reminded of Fritz Lang's memorable film, *Metropolis*. The shop windows were crammed with goods and with the artificial means to quell despair, and yet there was an air of unbearable loneliness everywhere. It was reflected in the numb, shut-in expressions of the people hurrying by. How many of them were on their way home to an empty flat or a lonely marriage? For all its wealth, the western world is inhabited by millions who are spiritually utterly bereft.

'Those who are disobedient' are those who ignore real wealth when they are offered it, for the riches which are really worth having are not for us to take or to work for, but rather to wait for, as a great unconditional gift from the Giver of Life. Every single person who has experienced Christ as a reality in their lives is the richest person on earth, whose personal wealth makes the sum of all the contents of all the shops in Oxford Street amount to no more than a handful of Christmas cracker trinkets.

In Christ we are both rich and truly alive. He has bequeathed to us his living presence. All that are required of us are pure and open hearts disposed to receiving his great bequest and to passing it on to the world in the way in which we live our lives and relate to others.

Action

Take into your heart the face of an anonymous passer-by and imagine that person enfolded in the love of God's Holy Spirit.

Quinguagesima Sunday
Seventh before Easter

Reading

If I speak in the tongues of mortals and of angels, but do not have love, I am a noisy gong or a clanging cymbal. And if I have prophetic powers, and understand all mysteries and all knowledge, and if I have all faith, so as to remove mountains, but do not have love, I am nothing. If I give away all my possessions, and if I hand over my body so that I may boast, but do not have love, I gain nothing.

Love is patient; love is kind; love is not envious or boastful or arrogant or rude. It does not insist on its own way; it is not irritable or resentful; it does not rejoice in wrongdoing, but rejoices in the truth. It bears all things, believes all things, hopes all things, endures all things.

Love never ends. But as for prophecies, they will come to an end; as for tongues, they will cease; as for knowledge, it will come to an end. For we know only in part, and we prophecy only in part; but when the complete comes, the partial will come to an end. When I was a child, I spoke like a child, I thought like a child, I reasoned like a child; when I became an adult, I put an end to childish ways. For now we see in a mirror, dimly, but then we will see face to face. Now I know only in part; then I will know fully, even as I have been fully known. And now faith, hope and love abide, these three; and the greatest of these is love (1 Cor. 13 NRSV).

Meditation

We are reminded before the beginning of Lent that the things which are not done in compassion towards neighbour and towards self are utterly meaningless. Self-denial which is not grounded in real love for God, and which does not spring from a genuine desire to be changed by him into a new person, is no more than a sort of spiritual obstacle course. It can only end in smug self-satisfaction or in a sense of futility and failure.

Love is the essence of creativity. The period which we are about to embark on is a kind of springtime of the soul, a time of growth and renewal which is wrought on us by Christ himself through our loving acquiescence to the action of his Holy Spirit dwelling in us. Furthermore, our capacity for love, and with it for knowing God, must extend to all people and to all creation, for the covenant of God's love, given in the rainbow and affirmed in the Cross, exists not only for our individual benefit, but that we might also be a part of his plan for loving the world to Salvation.

Action

It is customary among Jewish people to begin Yom Kippur, the Jewish Day of Atonement, by seeking the forgiveness of anyone whom one has wronged or offended during the year. It would be a good thing if between now and Ash Wednesday we were to seek out any member of our household (or any other person for that matter) whom we may have wronged in some way, and make our peace with them.

Shrove Tuesday

Reading

He went out again beside the sea; and all the crowd gathered about him, and he taught them. And as he passed on, he saw Levi the son of Alphaeus sitting at the tax office, and he said to him, 'Follow me.' And he rose and followed him.

And as he sat at table in his house, many tax collectors and sinners were sitting with Jesus and his disciples; for there were many who followed him. And the scribes of the Pharisees, when they saw that he was eating with sinners and tax collectors, said to his disciples, 'Why does he eat with tax collectors and sinners?' And when Jesus heard it, he said to them, 'Those who are well have no need of a physician, but those who are sick; I came not to call the righteous, but sinners' (Mark 2:13–17).

Meditation

Lent is a period of focused discipleship. It is a time set apart from the rest of the year so that we may concentrate on our Christian discipleship, as individuals and as the corporate body of Christ in the Church. This discipleship means treading whatever path happens to be open to us at any given moment in our lives – in other words it means being faithful to Christ in whatever circumstances we find ourselves.

We are not at the same point on our spiritual journey as we were this time a year ago, any more than we are at the same point in all the practical circumstances of our lives. Things have happened to us. We may be richer or poorer. We may have changed jobs, moved house, got married or ended a relationship. We are different people and the path which we tread will be in some measure different to the one trodden last year.

The path of discipleship, and particularly the Lenten one, is an invitation to a renewal of the whole person. It is a time when Christ comes to sit and eat with those who recognise their need for him. Lent is a season of growth and of growing in awareness and desire for God, rather than one of gratuitous and often wholly arbitrary acts of self-denial. It is in fact a journey of discovery, an occasion for the sort of deep and steady joy which wells up from the peace of a heart centred in its desire to know, love and serve God fully. Let this pure and simple desire be the one which takes precedence over every other consideration this Lent. Be prepared for the unexpected – and be prepared for sudden joy.

Action

Here is a pancake recipe with which to celebrate the joy which lies ahead in the coming weeks:

INGREDIENTS

$\frac{1}{2}$lb plain flour
2 standard eggs
1 pint milk
$\frac{1}{4}$tsp salt
Oil for cooking

Sieve the flour and salt into a mixing bowl and make a well in the middle of the flour. Into this break the eggs and mix gradually with a wooden spoon, adding half the milk and drawing in the flour. When this is smoothly mixed, beat it vigorously for 5–10 minutes to introduce plenty of air. Cover the bowl and leave to stand for 30–60 minutes in a cool place. At the end of that time, gently stir in the remaining milk and transfer the mixture to a jug.

In a frying pan, briskly heat a little oil and when it is smoking, pour into it sufficient batter mixture to cover the base of the pan thinly. Cook until the underside of the pancake is browned, then turn it over with a wide fish slice. When the second side is brown, slide the pancake on to a wire cake rack.

Continue to cook pancakes until batter mixture is used, adding a little *hot* oil to the pan as necessary. Stack the pancakes, after each one is cooked, interleaved with grease-proof paper.

The traditional English way to serve pancakes on Shrove Tuesday is sprinkled with sugar and lemon juice.

LENT

Ash Wednesday

Reading

'Yet even now,' says the Lord, 'return to me with all your heart, with fasting, with weeping, and with mourning; and rend your hearts and not your garments.' Return to the Lord, your God, for he is gracious and merciful, slow to anger, and abounding in steadfast love, and repents of evil (Joel 2:12–13).

Meditation

God meets us in Christ who rescues us from far-off places and who turns back with us towards home. Christ 'repents of evil' on our behalf in taking upon himself the inevitable consequences of our hardness of heart.

We live in a loveless world which, for the most part, goes its own way in blindness and obstinacy, in its refusal to recognise the action of a loving God, much less to invite him into its affairs. As a result of this, the gate to Heaven has become clogged with weeds and with the sort of dank undergrowth which only grows in dark and unhealthy places. It has been made narrow as the eye of a needle. Into this depressing situation comes Christ crucified who tears down the tangled undergrowth and makes the entrance wide for us, so that this very day, by even the smallest loving response to his call, we can be with him in Paradise.

Fasting is not so much a matter of 'giving things up for Lent' as of looking into our inner selves to see what areas need to be cut down so that new growth can take place. Any act of self-denial, any form of giving, will then be an affirmation and a celebration of the rending of our hearts and of God's living presence with us.

Action

Here are some suggestions for fasting and giving which focus on the renewal of the inner person. As they do not involve food and drink, they are ideal for people who lead busy and demanding lives.

SUGGESTIONS FOR GIVING
Live the virtue you most need –
   live humbly, patiently, kindly, obediently, etc.

Be thoroughly joyful
   (which does not mean being superficially cheerful).

Make someone else happy by a visit, a phone call or a letter.

Plan each day to be at your spiritual best, so becoming
   a centre of spiritual health for others.

Be prepared to take really well the things which rub you
   up the wrong way.

Read a solid book or two.

SUGGESTIONS FOR FASTING
Avoid

Reading, meetings and amusements distracting you from prayer and from the spiritual work in hand.

Thoughts centring round yourself, especially those which foster vanity or a sense of self-importance.

Critical or unkind thoughts of others.

Harbouring anything to grumble about, to resent, or to make you touchy.

Expressing temper or irritation.

Gloomy and morbid thoughts.

Getting over-tired. (Live within your limits and practise moderation in all things.)

Weekdays following
Ash Wednesday
Thursday

Reading

Happy are those who do not follow the advice of the wicked,
or take the path that sinners tread,
or sit in the seat of scoffers;
but their delight is in the law of the Lord,
and on his law they meditate day and night.
They are like trees
planted by streams of water,
which yield their fruit in its season,
and their leaves do not wither.
In all that they do, they prosper.

The wicked are not so,
but are like chaff that the wind drives away.
Therefore the wicked will not stand in the judgment,
nor sinners in the congregation of the righteous,
for the Lord watches over the way of the righteous,
but the way of the wicked will perish (Ps. 1 NRSV).

Meditation

This psalm is a recipe for perfect happiness. Seeking God,
meditating on his law is not a matter of straining to be 'good',
but of waiting with glad anticipation, as a child waits for a

promised treat, for God to happen in and through us in unexpected ways. We are not to think of ourselves as programmed like robots, but as the children of a loving parent who have been endowed with will and desire, as a magnificent treat, that our days be made happy in harmonising our desires with the Father's design for the world and for our individual destiny.

Happy are those whose lives are not governed by fashion, whose tastes are not dictated by the media, or by their own social class, or even by the religious attitudes with which they have felt comfortable for years. Happy are those who dare to move on. Happy are those whose desire is not for the short-lived and vacuous prestige which comes from conforming to selfish standards, even though these may be 'politically correct'. Happy are those who resist the temptation to walk down the paths of current thinking, simply because it is current. Happy are those who, having committed their way to God, stand as persons in their own right and respect all people who speak the truth and behave with integrity. Happy are those who are able to discern the truth and proclaim it out of a pure heart in every walk of modern life. They are like trees planted by streams of water . . . in all that they do they prosper, for inwardly they are at peace with God.

Action

We are to be known by the fruits we bear. Examine your priorities and politics, as well as old and possibly outdated opinions, and bring them up to date if necessary.

Friday

Reading

Those who are well have no need of a physician, but those who are sick; I came not to call the righteous, but sinners (Mark 2:17).

Meditation

Review briefly whatever came out of the meditation for Septuagesima Sunday (p.60).

We are as much involved in the sins of the world and of our society as we are in our own. Society's sins can make us feel spiritually ill. Whether we like it or not we, as individuals in the west, have a share in the collective sin of greed and selfishness which causes wars, famine and the destruction and waste of our environment. The solution lies neither in trying to shift the blame or in giving up in despair when faced with the futility of taking on the mega-rich and powerful bodies that seem to control the world's destiny.

The healing and forgiveness offered by Christ in every situation are those of transformation. It is the transforming of the cruel and the ugly into a new creation, not by our lone efforts, but by our desire that the world be conformed to his will and to his image. This desire lives in the heart of every person who is willing to give the time and take a little of the world's suffering to the one who has the power both to heal and to forgive. The world is held together by this kind of intercessory prayer.

Action

Read the newspaper or watch the news and draw the world
situation and the politics of the day into your own conscious
need for Christ's healing.

Saturday

Reading

If you take away from the midst of
you the yoke,
the pointing of the finger, and
speaking wickedness,
if you pour yourself out for the hungry
and satisfy the desire of the afflicted,
then shall your light rise in the darkness
and your gloom be as the noonday.
And the Lord will guide you continually,
and satisfy your desire with good things,
and make your bones strong;
and you shall be like a watered garden,
like a spring of water,
whose waters fail not
(Isa. 58:9b–11).

Meditation

Lent is a time of setting one's house to rights, of examining small everyday things, so that through them we can reorder our lives. It is also a time to make sure that whatever happens in prayer is reflected by our actions. Am I overbearing with my children? Critical and judgmental of others? Am I fully present to another person's need, giving them my full attention and, if called upon, the best of my time?

In order to find fulfilment, we do not seek an abstract 'out there' kind of God, but the reality of the living God encountered in the immediate and the ordinary.

Action

Reserve ten to fifteen minutes during the day for the following exercise. It need not always be done at night, but it should be done at the end of a twenty-four hour period:

1 Be relaxed and ask God for the grace to allow your whole being to be directed to his praise and service.

2 Let the day play back to you in any order and relish the moments you have enjoyed. Be thankful for them because they are God's gift to you.

3 Without judging yourself, look at your moods, attitudes and reactions to other people and situations and ask yourself – is everything that I do done out of a love for God and a desire to serve him, or are the things that I do really for my own glory and benefit?

4 Ask God for the grace to feel sorry for those times when you have failed to respond to him in the events of the day and know that his forgiveness is never withheld. Feel glad and grateful for the times when you have responded to him.

5 Ask for his guidance for tomorrow and allow him into all that you hope of it.

This exercise, known as the Examen of Consciousness, forms part of the Ignatian Spiritual Exercises, but it is an excellent habit for anyone to acquire and, if possible, to keep for life.

Saint David
1 March

Reading

The man who fears the Lord will do this, and he who holds to the law will obtain wisdom. She will come to meet him like a mother, and like the wife of his youth she will welcome him. She will feed him with the bread of understanding, and give him the water of wisdom to drink. He will lean on her and will not fall, and he will rely on her and will not be put to shame. She will exalt him above his neighbours, and will open his mouth in the midst of the assembly (Sirach 15:1–6).

Meditation

Saint David is thought of as the spiritual father of Wales. He is remembered for founding an order of monks on the site of the present cathedral of Saint David and for the wisdom and holiness of his life.

Wisdom is embodied in the word 'understanding' which also means to go with or to feel for, as with compassion. Wisdom is therefore inextricably bound up in compassion. The kind of wisdom which comes to people who lead holy lives is not necessarily intellectual, although it can be that as well. It is rather an instinct for the truth and empathy with people and with animals. 'Give me understanding that I may keep thy law' (Ps. 119:34) is the prayer of David, the psalmist. The law of life as given to us by Christ replaces all forms of legalism – rigid and impossible rules which do nothing to mould a person's heart and personality into an image of the divine Creator. The law of which David speaks, and which is kept by the wise, is a gift – the result of Christ's keeping of the old law to perfection on our behalf. To be wise is to live with this understanding so that it underpins our lives. In a world of confusing and conflicting values where we are always running the risk of compromising ourselves, we badly need this kind of wisdom that we may be alive in the fullest sense of the word.

Action

If you are involved in any kind of committee, resolve to speak up for wise and compassionate decisions rather than settling for the merely cost-effective and expedient.

First Sunday in Lent

Reading

Jesus, full of the Holy Spirit, returned from the Jordan, and was led by the Spirit for forty days in the wilderness, tempted by the devil. And he ate nothing in those days; and when they were ended, he was hungry. The devil said to him, 'If you are the Son of God, command this stone to become bread.' And Jesus answered him, 'It is written, "Man shall not live by bread alone."' And the devil took him up, and showed him all the kingdoms of the world in a moment of time, and said to him, 'To you I will give all this authority and their glory; for it has been delivered to me, and I give it to whom I will. If you, then, will worship me, it shall all be yours.' And Jesus answered him, 'It is written, "You shall worship the Lord your God, and him only shall you serve."'

And he took him to Jerusalem, and set him on the pinnacle of the temple, and said to him, 'If you are the Son of God, throw yourself down from here; for it is written, "He will give his angels charge of you, to guard you," and "On their hands they will bear you up, lest you strike your foot against a stone."' And Jesus answered him, 'It is said, "You shall not tempt the Lord your God."' And when the devil had ended every temptation, he departed from him until an opportune time (Luke. 4:1–13).

Meditation

Christ goes ahead to meet us in every form of testing. These temptations are as real as our own. They are as real as the moment when we are on the very brink of having or doing the one thing we had promised ourselves not to have or do. Temptation is always a threshold, a cliff edge situation, because all of a sudden the thing which we deny ourselves is within easy reach, and the denying of it, in the broad light of day seems ludicrous. It must have seemed so to Jesus who was not only faint with hunger, but perhaps felt that the task of laying down his life literally, as well as in the daily dying to his rightful glory, was, after all, ludicrous and unnecessary.

The devil is called the prince of lies because, in his anthropomorphised form, he is an expert in the empty and counterfeit, and in the things of the world. In this respect, power, success, glory and wealth are indeed his to give. The wilderness of the spirit is not only a place where we are invited for no apparent reason to give way to rather mundane temptations, but a colourless wasteland of shrivelled dreams, where God seems never to have existed. The main temptation lies in believing that what we know to be true is, in fact, a lie and with filling the yawning vacuum which this creates with anything that comes to mind. Faced with desolation we run for noise and distraction to help us put on a new face and disown the pain and the outrage. For this reason Jesus refuses Satan's offers but stands in his wilderness, owning the pain and uncertainty, that we might suddenly come across him in our time of testing and own his peace and his strength.

Action

If you are keeping a journal, read over what you wrote on Ash Wednesday and re-experience the positive feelings which were yours when you decided on your course for Lent. Ask God to be with you and to strengthen you in moments of temptation.

First Week in Lent
Monday

Reading

Say to all the congregation of the people of Israel, you shall be holy; for I the Lord your God am holy (Lev. 19:2).

Meditation

The real meaning of holiness is 'wholeness' – in other words the spiritual health which comes with being a complete person. Holiness is not a sublime state of consciousness reserved for people with esoteric interests, neither is it the special domain of those who have been chosen for the religious life; as if for some reason ordinary people who desire wholeheartedly to know God better and to be like him are being arrogant or presumptuous. There is no such thing as a 'professional' Christian, or for that matter, a 'professional' Buddhist, Jew or Moslem. Holiness is every person's birthright. The purpose of Lent is for us to claim that right, not by putting ourselves through a series of spiritual gymnastics, but by a simple desire to meet and release the captive Christ in ourselves and in others.

Action

Accomplish something today, no matter how small, in such a way that the action is whole or complete. You could try writing a letter which you have been putting off, thereby making whole something which was started some time ago.

The same thing applies to tidying out a cupboard, or cleaning the car or even taking the family dog for a long-overdue visit to the vet.

First Week in Lent
Tuesday

Reading

I sought the Lord, and he answered me,
and delivered me from all my fears.
Look to him, and be radiant;
so your faces shall never be ashamed.

Evil shall slay the wicked;
and those who hate the righteous will be condemned.
The Lord redeems the life of his servants;
none of those who take refuge in him will be condemned
(Ps. 34:4–5, 21,22).

Meditation

In today's world being 'condemned' is most likely to mean being made to feel a fool. We seek and desire God in the sure knowledge that he will never betray our trust by making fools of us. Those who 'condemn' or make fools of others because of their integrity are usually the ones who are made to feel most vulnerable by the 'righteousness' of those same people.

We seek and take refuge in God by daring to stand up for what we know to be righteous, in relationships, in politics and in the resolving of our own inner conflicts. This does not mean feeling smug or pious, but rather facing up to fear and to the uncompromising commitment of the heart and will which is required in Christian discipleship.

Re-read this passage slowly, allowing the things for which

you or someone known to you are unjustly 'condemned' to surface. Try not to let feelings of self-righteousness take over but forgive those who do the condemning from that place of strength which is yours – the abiding presence of the Lord.

Action

Write a letter to a newspaper supporting the actions of anyone in public life who is behaving with integrity and courage, especially if their behaviour is unpopular with the majority. Support a friend or neighbour, or a relative who may be suffering for 'righteousness' sake'.

First Week in Lent
Wednesday

Reading

The sacrifice acceptable to God is a broken spirit;
a broken and contrite heart, O God, thou wilt not despise
(Ps. 51:17).

Meditation

These words are not addressed to an angry and vengeful deity, who desires nothing better than to see his victims squirm with humiliation. On the contrary, they reflect God's yearning to be in intimate union with us. In order for this union to be realised, it is necessary that we become broken down, as the bread of the Eucharist is broken in commemoration of the broken body of Christ. Being inwardly broken is essential if we are to be co-mingled with God as the water and the wine are co-mingled at that same Eucharist. It is not a matter of being beaten or cowed into submission, but of being pliant and willing to move with God in a joyful celebration and response to his love for us and for all creation.

Action

Be aware of how much more manageable a thing is when it is broken up into pieces. You can do this exercise when slicing a loaf of bread, or cutting up some vegetables, or sawing a piece of wood.

First Week in Lent
Thursday

Reading

Ask, and it will be given you; search, and you will find; knock, and the door will be opened for you. For everyone who asks receives, and everyone who searches finds, and for everyone who knocks the door will be opened. Is there anyone among you who, if your child asks for bread, will give a stone? Or if the child asks for a fish, will give a snake? If you then, who are evil, know how to give good gifts to your children, how much more will your Father in heaven give good things to those who ask him! (Matt. 7:7–11 NRSV).

Meditation

Jesus is particularly concerned with the 'good things' which are ours for the asking. This does not mean unnecessary indulgences like giving sweets to spoilt children, but things which are really going to do us good, in the sense that they will make us more whole – more holy. They are therefore not necessarily the things which we think will be good for us. In fact, they may not even feel like gifts at all.

Suffering, no matter how trivial it may seem, is itself a mysterious gift because it has the potential for making us more like Christ and more fully united to him. For example, a person could ask for the grace (the 'good thing') to go without tea or coffee for a day, out of a loving desire to be in solidarity with Christ who fasted for forty days, as well as with those who, in our own times, experience hunger and deprivation.

The 'good thing' might manifest itself in a profound joy and even in a sense of God's own gratitude to us for undertaking this small but important act of self-denial. It may come as a complete surprise, an added bonus to what one was asking for or expecting.

Action

Do you find it difficult to ask for help or receive a favour? Make a point of letting someone know you need them today.

First Week in Lent
Friday

Reading

Bless the Lord, my soul, remembering all he has done for thee: he restores thy youth as the eagle's plumage is restored (Ps. 103:2,5).   Offertory.

Meditation

Lent is a time for renewal. It is also a time for realising that true joy, like the rarest and most precious of jewels, is often to be found at the heart of the painful process of our own inner renewal. Suffering and joy are inextricably linked in the person of Christ who is at one with us and with our present situation.

When a house is turned inside out so that it can be thoroughly cleaned, it seems to know that in due course order will be restored to it and its ruffled plumage will be made smooth and shining. The upheaval will have been worth it. Lent is a time of inner spring-cleaning and upheaval. When the upheaval seems more than we can bear and that we shall never be our 'old selves' again, it is sometimes helpful to remember all the things during the past year which have been a cause for joy and to try to give thanks for them. This little exercise helps one to keep things in perspective and prevents circumstances from overpowering us.

It is said that all of heaven rejoices over the repentance of one person who realises that they are on the wrong path, but it is equally true of the one who remembers life's blessings and gives thanks for them in the midst of tribulation.

Action

When you are doing your review of the day, pay special attention to those things for which you can be grateful and perceive in them your youth and plumage being restored.

Make a start on the spring cleaning, or on setting the garden to rights before the onset of the growing season, or sort through some long-neglected pile of papers. Brush the dog. Groom a horse.

First Week in Lent
Saturday

Reading

*You have heard that it was said, 'You shall love your neighbour
and hate your enemy.' But I say to you, Love your enemies and
pray for those who persecute you, so that you may be children of
your Father in heaven; for he makes his sun rise on the evil and on
the good, and sends rain on the righteous and on the unrighteous.
For if you love those who love you, what reward do you have? Do
not even the tax collectors do the same? And if you greet only your
brothers and sisters, what more are you doing than others? Do not
even the Gentiles do the same? Be perfect, therefore, as your
heavenly Father is perfect* (Matt. 5:43–end NRSV).

Meditation

In loving we are most closely united to God and with him to
the whole continuing process of creation. For love, like the
creative act itself, is first a matter of allowing and of letting be,
of not getting in the way of the work. The same is true in our
dealings with people, for every individual is a work of art, so
we love others by allowing these works of art to become fully
what God intends them to be. The allowing has to happen
even at a cost to ourselves, for love, like art, is full of risk.

All life is a learning process, a school for growing in the love
of God. This is as true of nations as it is for individuals. We
actively give space to young nations to take root and develop,
even though we in the more affluent countries may sometimes
feel threatened by them.

The power of the Christian message lies in the seeming foolishness of love freely given.

Action

Find a moment today to give space in your heart, where you meet and are united with Christ, for a person who has hurt you or for a nation or group of people with whom you feel uncertain.

The Holy Forty Martyrs
of Sebaste, AD 320
10 March

Reading

The fear of the Lord is the beginning of knowledge;
fools despise wisdom and instruction.
Hear, my child, your father's instruction,
and do not reject your mother's teaching;
for they are a fair garland for your head,
and pendants for your neck.
My child, if sinners entice you,
do not consent

(Prov. 1:7–11).

From the readings chosen for
Vespers in the Orthodox Church

Meditation

During the reign of the emperor Lucinius of Armenia, forty of
his soldiers refused to worship the pagan gods of the time and
defected to the Christian faith. As a punishment, Lucinius,
who was renowned for his cruelty, ordered that the soldiers be
stripped and tied to stakes set into the ice of a frozen lake and
there left to die. In addition to this, he provided them with an
added incentive for a change of heart in the shape of a warm
fire and a hot bath on the nearby shore. When one of them
relented a soldier on guard duty was so touched by the courage

and innocence of the man's companions that he threw off his clothes and rushed to take his place.

Martyrdom of this sort is not often called for today, but a daily and continuous owning of our allegiance to Christ is most certainly demanded of Christians in the modern world. Be aware then of those moments when we are all challenged on what we stand for. Is our Christian faith merely a set of morals or a cosy and 'personal' spirituality, or does our love for Christ overflow in continuous and often unconscious desire for people in the world to realise their union with him?

Action

Have a look at the baptism service which is usually printed on a card and available in most churches. It is customary to renew these vows at Easter, so think about their relevance for your life today. If the language seems remote you could try writing out a modern version, so that you can renew your vows privately (or in the company of others) on Easter Sunday.

Second Sunday in Lent

Reading

There is therefore now no condemnation for those who are in Christ Jesus (Rom. 8:1).

Meditation

No condemnation – no blame. In Christ we are made innocent. In Christ we live our whole lives as though we stood before him in an eternal present moment of reconciliation. While desiring for this state of being to remain unspoiled, we do nothing in our own strength because everything is done in us and through us.

We are on a journey like that of Alice and the Red Queen, constantly arriving at our destination while simultaneously pressing forward to reach it. But unlike Alice and the Queen, who ran their fastest without covering any ground at all, we do not push and strain in our own strength but move with the rhythm of God's own music, available to his love, open and allowing to his will. There can therefore be no condemnation for those who journey through life in this way – no risk of disappointing God by failing to meet a particular set of standards, no wasting of personal resources and no taking advantage of our weakness, for God does not play games with the emotions of those who trust him.

Action

As a celebration of our freedom from blame, a good Sunday tea would be in order. Here is a recipe for hot cross buns:

INGREDIENTS

450g (1lb) strong plain flour
1 pkt dry yeast
1 level tsp salt
½ level tsp each of mixed spice, powdered cinnamon, grated
    nutmeg
50g (2oz) caster sugar
50g (2oz) butter, melted and cooled, but not firm
1 egg, beaten
100/125g (4oz) currants
25–50g (1–2oz) chopped mixed peel

For the glaze
4 tbsp milk and water
40g (1½ oz) castor sugar

Flour a baking sheet. Prepare the dry yeast according to the manufacturer's instructions and set aside until it is frothy. This will take anything up to 45 minutes, depending on room temperature. Sift together the remaining flour, the salt, spices and 50g sugar. Stir the butter and egg into the frothy yeast mixture, add the spiced flour and the fruit, and mix together. The dough should be fairly soft but not sticky. Turn it out on to a lightly floured surface and knead until smooth and malleable. Leave to rise until doubled in size – about 1–1½ hours. Again, this will depend on room temperature. Turn the risen dough out on to a floured surface and knock out the air bubbles, then knead.

Divide the dough into 12 pieces and shape into buns, using the palm of one hand. Press down hard at first on the table surface, then ease up as you turn and shape the buns. Arrange them well apart on the floured baking sheet, and prove for about 45 minutes (only 30 minutes if the dough has had an initial rising). Make quick slashes with a very sharp knife or razor, just cutting the surface of the dough, to make a cross. Bake just above the centre of a fairly hot oven (375°F, gas mark 5) for 15–20 minutes. Brush the hot buns twice with glaze, then leave to cool.

Second Week in Lent
Monday

Reading

He also told this parable to some who trusted in themselves that they were righteous and despised others: 'Two men went up into the temple to pray, one a Pharisee and the other a tax collector. The Pharisee stood and prayed thus with himself, "God, I thank thee that I am not like other men, extortioners, unjust, adulterers, or even like this tax collector. I fast twice a week, I give tithes of all that I get." But the tax collector, standing far off, would not even lift up his eyes to heaven, but beat his breast, saying "God, be merciful to me a sinner!" I tell you, this man went down to his house justified rather than the other; for every one who exalts himself will be humbled, but he who humbles himself will be exalted' (Luke 18:9–15).

Meditation

A devout Christian goes into a cathedral with the intention of spending twenty minutes or so in one of the side chapels. She passes by the large box with a notice above it specifying a minimum donation towards the upkeep of the building. She makes a mental note of the fact that she has come to pray and is therefore exempt from having to make donations. She also unconsciously laments the tramping of feet, the screaming children and the guided tours, as well as the whistles and shouts of builders working on scaffolding in the chancel. She is grateful that she is not a mere tourist, insensitive to the real purpose and meaning of this place. She also feels that the

98

builders should work quietly and moderate their language in what is, after all, a church. On her way out, however, she notices that one of the Americans, a rather florid gentleman, festooned in cameras and clearly suffering from the heat (it is a sweltering day in mid August) has sat down in front of the statue of the Virgin who is holding the Christ-child. He is mopping his brow and simply looking at the Child who returns his gaze with a smile and a greeting. As she is about to leave she passes one of the builders who is meticulously removing some dust which has fallen on one of the carvings near where he had been working. He does this with reverence and affection.

Real humility lies in recognising with gratitude the gifts which one has been given without judging or presuming on the moral or spiritual state of other people.

Action

If there is a cathedral or old church near you, spend some time enjoying the building for its own sake and be aware of God's love for all those who visit it.

Second Week in Lent
Tuesday

Reading

When Jesus had thus spoken, he was troubled in spirit, and testified, 'Truly, truly, I say to you, one of you will betray me.' The disciples looked at one another, uncertain of whom he spoke. One of his disciples, whom Jesus loved, was lying close to the breast of Jesus; so Simon Peter beckoned to him and said, 'Tell us who it is of whom he speaks.' So lying thus, close to the breast of Jesus, he said to him, 'Lord, who is it?' Jesus answered, 'It is he to whom I shall give this morsel when I have dipped it.' So when he had dipped the morsel, he gave it to Judas, the son of Simon Iscariot.

Then after the morsel, Satan entered into him. Jesus said to him, 'What you are going to do, do quickly.' Now no one at the table knew why he said this to him. Some thought that, because Judas had the money box, Jesus was telling him, 'Buy what we need for the feast'; or, that he should give something to the poor. So, after receiving the morsel, he immediately went out; and it was night (John 13:21–30).

Meditation

Judas was a man with a dream. His impatience, and possibly his desire to be proved right, drove him to set up a situation whose outcome would be the realisation of that dream. Perhaps, as a disciple, he felt frustrated and disillusioned in his calling – others were obviously more popular than he was – or perhaps he simply felt taken for granted. He may have been a rather colourless character and envied Peter for his charismatic personality. In any case, despite his position of responsibility, he seems to have had some sort of a chip on his shoulder.

Whatever was the cause of his inferiority complex, he was prepared to risk the life of the one person he loved in order to justify himself. Viewed in this context, Judas seems to be taking upon himself the responsibility for the work of redemption, as though Jesus has somehow got it wrong. He may have meant well. He may also have believed that Jesus was bluffing when he spoke of the suffering he was to endure and that he would extricate himself at the last minute. But whatever was going through his mind at the time, Judas was human.

There is a Judas in all of us, full of self-doubt, capable of making the most appalling misjudgments, capable of betrayal in its subtlest forms, capable of panic and despair. This is the Judas whom we must learn to love and forgive.

Action

If you have betrayed someone in any way, do something, no matter how small, to put it right.

Second Week in Lent
Wednesday

Reading

And as Jesus was going up to Jerusalem, he took the twelve disciples aside, and on the way he said to them, 'Behold, we are going up to Jerusalem; and the Son of man will be delivered to the chief priests and scribes and they will condemn him to death, and deliver him to the Gentiles to be mocked and scourged and crucified, and he will be raised on the third day.'

Then the mother of the sons of Zebedee came up to him, with her sons, and kneeling before him she asked him for something. And he said to her, 'What do you want?' She said to him, 'Command that these two sons of mine may sit, one at your right hand and one at your left, in your kingdom.' But Jesus answered, 'You do not know what you are asking. Are you able to drink the cup that I am to drink?' They said to him, 'We are able.' He said to them, 'You will drink my cup, but to sit at my right hand and at my left is not mine to grant, but it is for those for whom it has been prepared by my Father.' And when the ten heard it they were indignant at the two brothers. But Jesus called them to him and said, 'You know that the rulers of the Gentiles lord it over them, and their great men exercise authority over them. It shall not be so among you; but whoever would be great among you must be your servant, and whoever would be first among you must be your slave; even as the Son of man came not to be served but to serve, and to give his life as a ransom for many (Matt. 20:17–28).

Meditation

Everyone knows what it feels like when one has something important to say and nobody appears to be listening, or else someone abruptly changes the subject.

Experience, in reading this passage, not only the sense of rejection which Christ experienced, but also the sense of futility which must have accompanied it. How, even at this stage, did he find the courage to persevere in what he had been sent to do? It could only have been possible through a reckless and uncompromising love towards those around him, a love which was extended to the whole human race throughout all time.

Jesus is not driven to irritability by the mother and her two sons, neither does he try to embarrass them by lecturing them on humility. The sense of outrage comes from the other disciples. Instead, Jesus counsels them all, with the utmost courtesy, to grow in compassion, in the desire to be given over out of love to the service of others.

Humility is the fruit of compassion. The realisation, the consciousness of our union with Christ, is expressed in the desire to serve creation and all living beings.

Action

Make a point of serving someone today by listening 'underneath' what they are saying, thereby identifying with their pain and with their need for love. The greatest gift we can give another person is our full and undivided attention and unlimited space in our own inner being.

Second Week in Lent
Thursday

Reading

There was a rich man, who was clothed in purple and fine linen and who feasted sumptuously every day. And at his gate lay a poor man named Lazarus, full of sores, who desired to be fed with what fell from the rich man's table; moreover the dogs came and licked his sores. The poor man died and was carried by the angels to Abraham's bosom. The rich man also died and was buried; and in Hades, being in torment, he lifted up his eyes, and saw Abraham far off and Lazarus in his bosom. And he called out, 'Father Abraham, have mercy upon me, and send Lazarus to dip the end of his finger in water and cool my tongue; for I am in anguish in this flame.' But Abraham said, 'Son, remember that you in your lifetime received your good things, and Lazarus in like manner evil things; but now he is comforted here, and you are in anguish. And besides all this, between us and you a great chasm has been fixed, in order that those who would pass from here to you may not be able, and none may cross from there to us.' And he said, 'Then I beg you, father, to send him to my father's house, for I have five brothers, so that he may warn them, lest they also come into this place of torment.' But Abraham said, 'They have Moses and the prophets; let them hear them.' And he said, 'No, father Abraham; but if some one goes to them from the dead, they will repent.' He said to him, 'If they do not hear Moses and the prophets, neither will they be convinced if some one should rise from the dead' (Luke 16:19–end).

Meditation

It seems hard to believe that a person with even a grain of compassion could be confined to hell for all time. Perhaps a sort of clearing-house exists where, at some cost, we are made fit to spend eternity in the company of the angels. This particular 'place of torment' might be called purgatory.

Hell is by definition anti-life and I, for one, would like to believe that as a unique and permanent fixture it is quite inconsistent with the notion of the all-powerful God of Love. How the God of infinite love reconciles the need for infinite justice is something which is beyond the scope of human understanding. However, whatever we believe about hell and purgatory, there certainly exists a place where people who do not accept God's invitation to love life in the fullest sense of the word may well end up, at least for a period of finite time.

The Lazarus story is therefore a cautionary tale in not presuming that all will automatically be well, as long as we are at least loyal to our own kin. It points to the fact that we are every bit as related to the stranger in any kind of need (not only financial) as we are to members of our own family, and that the penalty for ignoring this law of love could be severe. But Christ has visited and claimed dominion over hell, so that even this realm of darkness is his and must ultimately be redeemed by him.

Action

Make a little space in your heart for anyone known to you who has died. Do this without passing judgment on their lives and try to forgive them for any wrong they may have done you. Let the hurt be, and really wish them well with your whole heart. This is a way of responding to the request from Dives, the rich man in torment, for water to slake his thirst.

If you have a friend or a relative who is buried near where you live, go and place some spring flowers on their grave.

Second Week in Lent
Friday

Reading

Therefore the Lord himself will give you a sign. Behold, a young woman shall conceive and bear a son, and shall call his name Emmanuel (Isa. 7:14).

From the Orthodox Liturgy of the Presanctified Gifts
Friday of the second week of Great Lent

Meditation

Lent is a time of travelling towards Holy Week and the ultimate sacrifice of Calvary, but in times of darkness and difficulty we are reminded that the Cross itself is a sign of hope and that Christ our Emmanuel is with us at the heart of every present moment.

The name Emmanuel means 'God with us'. We carry Christ as Mary carried him by 'couching' him in our hearts. 'Couching' is a Welsh expression meaning to hold a child close to one's body. Usually the mother and child are enfolded in a single shawl. So in prayer we enfold Christ in his suffering and Christ, the child, in all his vulnerability. Saint Veronica's action of wiping the face of the suffering Christ was an act of 'couching' which was rewarded by his gift to her of the imprint of his features on the linen which she had used to minister to him. It was the first icon and the name, Veronica, means 'true icon'.

Try to 'couch' Christ in your heart in your time of prayer. If you find it helpful, pray with an icon of the Virgin and child, or with a painting which allows you to cherish and hold the suffering Christ, and with him all of creation.

Action

Do someone a favour, and in the doing of it cherish the person you are serving.

Second Week in Lent
Saturday

Reading

It was fitting to make merry and be glad, for this your brother was dead, and is alive; he was lost, and is found (Luke 15:32).

Meditation

Repentance – finding the right road, coming home – is above all an occasion for celebration. The same is true for the healing of hurts and the resolving of differences between individuals and between nations. The paradox of the Christian life lies in the joy we experience as the outcome of suffering and out of conflict that has been consecrated in forgiveness. The hurts which we inflict on one another are transformed into something of infinite value when repentance and forgiveness are laid upon them.

The story of the prodigal son is about unconditional and reckless love, love that defies reason and common sense. Our response to Christ's invitation to go forward into the risky business of forgiveness has to be unconditional and reckless, as his love for us is unconditional and reckless. It is a matter of allowing, at great risk to ourselves, a situation which causes us pain, whether it is in a personal relationship or on an international scale, simply to be in Christ so that the pain in the situation, the person or the nation can be absorbed by him. Our relationship with that person, or group of people, or nation, undergoes with Christ a process of transfiguration and resurrection. The hurtful situation is wiped off the record. It is as though it had never existed in the first place.

We do not forgive and forget. Instead, we let go and allow for resurrection and new life to happen between us and those who have wronged us, so that a love which was lost is found, and our fear of other nations or people is transformed into hope and new life.

Action

Watch or listen to the news in silence and with a heart that is centred in the world's pain. If a state of conflict exists between nations or groups of people in society, or if some terrible crime has been committed, allow that situation simply to exist in your heart, in Christ. Cherish all the parties involved. Recognise with honesty that it is only by the love of God that you and I have been prevented, perhaps through no more than material circumstances, from going down a similar path.

Befriend someone with a difficult personality. If you know of someone in prison, make arrangement to visit them.

Third Sunday in Lent

Reading

The Lord said: 'I am the Lord your God, who brought you out of the land of Egypt, out of the house of bondage. You shall have no other gods before me. You shall not make for yourself a graven image, or any likeness of anything that is in heaven above, or that is on the earth beneath, or that is in the water under the earth; you shall not bow down to them or serve them ... You shall not take the name of the Lord your God in vain ... Observe the sabbath day, to keep it holy, as the Lord your God commanded you ... Honour your father and your mother, as the Lord your God commanded you, You shall not kill. Neither shall you commit adultery ... Neither shall you steal. Neither shall you bear false witness against your neighbour. Neither shall you covet anything that is your neighbour's' (Deut. 5:5–9, 11, 12, 16, 19–20, 21).

Meditation

The object of the commandments is not to suffocate and restrict, but to make us free to seek God. They are the equivalent of coloured cones put along a motorway, so that the traffic can proceed with reasonable speed towards its destination without getting mixed up with the road works, which would result in chaos and endanger life.

Seeking God in order to experience him (knowing God means experiencing him) is the whole purpose of our existence. The commandments are there as guidelines to help us to realise our union with God, the reality of the kingdom of

111

heaven within us. This kingdom of heaven is not a euphoric state of oblivion, neither is it some sort of superior 'consciousness', although it does involve being conscious of the reality of the living Christ present to our every present moment, the Christ whose resurrection is reflected in the life which surrounds us in the natural world and in our fellow human beings.

Action

Next time you find yourself in a traffic jam caused by road works, take the time to centre from the heart on the reality of Christ within you. This exercise is a very good antidote to stressful situations and works well when waiting in a queue, or when put on 'hold' during a telephone conversation.

Any kind of waiting is in itself a useful spiritual exercise. Use it to reinforce a sense of waiting on God for him to manifest himself to you in some surprising way.

Third Week in Lent
Monday

Reading

And Jesus said, 'Truly, I say to you, no prophet is acceptable in his own country. But in truth, I tell you, there were many widows in Israel in the days of Elijah, when the heaven was shut up three years and six months, when there came a great famine over all the land; and Elijah was sent to none of them but only to Zarephath, in the land of Sidon, to a woman who was a widow. And there were many lepers in Israel in the time of the prophet Elisha; and none of them was cleansed, but only Naaman the Syrian.' When they heard this, all in the synagogue were filled with wrath. And they rose up and put him out of the city, and led him to the brow of the hill on which their city was built, that they might throw him down headlong. But passing through the midst of them he went away (Luke 4:24–30).

Meditation

It is dangerous to presume that we are safe and earmarked for salvation merely because we call ourselves Christians. Just as there were many lepers who were not cleansed, so there are many nominal Christians, or even quite hearty ones, for that matter, who may fail to find what they expect at the end of life's journey. Nothing that we do of ourselves guarantees us any kind of passport to eternal life. With this in mind, it is easy to imagine how angry and threatened these religious experts felt when the truth of the words of Jesus dawned on them; that for all their expertise, they did not necessarily qualify for the kingdom of heaven. Even today as we approach the new millennium, the living reality of Emmanuel, God with us, lies quite outside such considerations. The less we are qualified, the more we are likely to find Christ.

Action

The highly placed members of the religious establishment were angry because their integrity was being challenged. Listen carefully to any opinion which may not coincide with yours and fully allow yourself to be challenged and even changed by it.

Third Week in Lent
Tuesday

Reading

Then Pharisees and scribes came to Jesus from Jerusalem and said, 'Why do your disciples transgress the tradition of the elders? For they do not wash their hands when they eat.' He answered them, 'And why do you transgress the commandment of God for the sake of your tradition? For God commanded, "Honour your father and your mother," and, "He who speaks evil of father or mother, let him surely die." But you say, "If anyone tells his father or his mother, What you would have gained from me is given to God, he need not honour his father." So, for the sake of your tradition, you have made void the word of God. You hypocrites! Well did Isaiah prophesy of you, when he said: "This people honours me with their lips, but their heart is far from me; in vain do they worship me, teaching as doctrines the precepts of men."' And he called the people to him and said to them, 'Hear and understand: not what goes into the mouth defiles a man, but what comes out of the mouth, this defiles a man' (Matt. 15:1–11).

Meditation

The meaning behind the symbol matters more than the symbol itself. Today, more than ever, it is important to learn to sit lightly to symbols and tradition, and instead to seek with our whole heart the living truth which they represent. Tradition is important insofar as it is observed with a loving heart and so fosters a still greater love for God, but it can very easily replace

God altogether. This is not to say that we should dispense with what is beautiful, because something that is truly beautiful (not just expertly made) can only be the product of love. With this in mind, our worship and our churches need to be made more beautiful; less functional perhaps, but more conducive to the lifting up of the eyes to behold and adore the present glory of God.

Turn to the action which accompanies this meditation and incorporate it into your prayer. Be ready to become centred into whatever you are doing at any point in the day so that the ordinary actions of everyday life become consecrated and an extension of your time of prayer.

Action

During the time you normally set aside for prayer, make something beautiful, purely out of love for God and as a gift for him. It could just as easily be a painting or a cake as a cleaned and polished car or flowers arranged with care.

Go to a church which you find pleasant to be in and enjoy its beauty, perceiving in it God's presence and perfection.

Third Week in Lent
Wednesday

Reading

Think not that I have come to abolish the law and the prophets; I have come not to abolish them but to fulfil them. For truly, I say to you, till heaven and earth pass away, not an iota, not a dot, will pass from the law until all is accomplished (Matt. 5:17–18).

Meditation

The purpose of 'the law' is to facilitate our experience of God. Just as the symbol encloses or represents the truth, so the 'law', the keeping of the commandments in spirit as well as in practice, slowly reveals and bequeaths to us an aspect of God's own beauty and perfection. We take possession of our inheritance of the kingdom of God within us by going forward to claim it in a wholehearted desire to live in the way God wants us to live. We seek and find him in our obedience to him in going with the ordinary and the present moment, rather than wishing and striving to be another person living in another place at some other point in time.

The 'law' is obedience or going with the present set of circumstances which we use creatively, in order to make something pleasing to the God whom we encounter hour by hour.

Action

Central to the life of many contemplative religious orders is the idea that work is prayer, so repeat yesterday's action by taking any one of the day's normal routine actions and make of it an offering to God as a loving fulfilment of the law. Activities which are particularly well suited to this kind of exercise include: washing up, laying a table, paying a bill, preparing food, feeding the family pets, etc.

Third Week in Lent
Thursday

Reading

Then Peter came up and said to him, 'Lord how often shall my brother sin against me, and I forgive him? As many as seven times?' Jesus said to him, 'I do not say to you seven times, but seventy times seven' (Matt. 18:21–2).

Meditation

The chief difficulty with forgiving a hurt done to one seems to lie with the fact that the hurt keeps coming back. It lives on as a memory. With the memory comes the temptation to 'unforgive' and to indulge in bitter and sometimes vengeful thoughts. It is all rather like a mosquito bite which if left alone will eventually disappear, while the smallest inadvertent scratch is enough to resuscitate it. Destructive thoughts have a way of creeping up on us even before we realise we are thinking them and with them returns the whole hurtful incident, twice as painful as it ever was in the first place.

The solution might be to treat the thoughts as we would treat an insect bite by first accepting that they exist, without hating them or ourselves in any way, and then applying soothing lotions, by thinking positively about the person in question (nobody is one hundred per cent bad after all!) and exercising the heart for all it is worth in genuinely desiring that person's well-being and happiness.

We need to forgive ourselves, too, for trying to make the forgiving of someone else a once and for all occurrence, so causing ourselves much unnecessary pain and guilt. Forgiveness is a continuous process without which growth cannot take place.

Action

Try writing a friendly letter (it doesn't have to be a long one) or making a quick telephone call to someone who really gets under your skin. Before doing this, though, use whatever means at your disposal to centre that person, and the action you are about to take, with you in Christ. In this way, it will be easier to draw on his resources to love and forgive the person from the heart (even if only for an hour or so) and to desire their happiness. Our own resources are quite inadequate when it comes to really forgiving someone.

Third Week in Lent
Friday

Reading

And he told this parable: 'A man had a fig tree planted in his vineyard; and he came seeking fruit on it and found none. And he said to the vinedresser, "Lo, these three years I have come seeking fruit on this fig tree, and I find none. Cut it down; why should it use up the ground?" And he answered him, "Let it alone, sir, this year also, till I dig about it and put on manure. And if it bears fruit next year, well and good; but if not, you can cut it down"' (Luke 13:6–9).

Meditation

We do not know the end of the story, but could it be that the fig-tree became more fruitful as a result of being let off?

Without forgiveness there can be no growth. Our treatment of the environment needs to be patterned on the way we ought to treat one another, for we are all part of one living organism which depends on love for its survival. The earth and its creatures depend, like us, on mutual patience and forgiveness, and on the loving discipline which we, as responsible vine-dressers, are able to give it.

Kindness to the earth and mercy on others are the central messages in this story but there is also a sombre note of warning. If next year, despite the vinedresser's gentle minis-trations, the tree does not bear fruit, it will be cut down (but not necessarily uprooted or killed). It is not for us to dispense judgment, only to help others realise their fullest potential while we look to our own growth, making sure that we continue to bear fruit.

If you are directly responsible for the growth of others, as a parent, teacher or employer, spend a little of this time reviewing to what extent you conscientiously and lovingly attend to their growth. How concerned are you about the whole of their existence, not just the part that directly affects you?

Action

If you have a garden, make sure that the land is in good heart by feeding it with manure or compost. Pay special attention to plants which need encouragement.

If you live in town, see to the well-being of any house plants which you may have. Some may need repotting, for example, or put fresh flowers in a room where they can be seen and enjoyed. Cut flowers thrive on appreciation.

Third Week in Lent
Saturday

Reading

Let us know, let us press on to know the Lord;
            his going forth is sure as the dawn;
he will come to us as the showers,
            as the spring rains that water the earth.

For I desire steadfast love and not sacrifice,
the knowledge of God, rather than burnt offerings
                                    (Hos. 6:3, 6).

Meditation

If you plant runner beans or french beans in a seed tray at this time of year, after a few days small mounds will begin to appear on the surface of the soil, followed by the beginnings of a new green shoot pressing its way out to the light. We too press our way out of darkness into the light of Christ. The bean knows, as only a bean can know, that it will be sure to find the light and moisture which it needs for its continued growth. In the same way, those who seek God from the heart can rest in the knowledge that all that they need for their spiritual growth will be provided for them.

A plant grows without thinking about growing. It does not strain to become something which it is not equipped to become. In the same way our own growth into the knowledge of God happens gently and imperceptibly. Knowledge of God means experience of him. It has nothing to do with intellectual ability, although we should use all the talents we are given, but stems from the desire of the heart for real relationship.

Action

Be ready for a surprise encounter with God at unexpected moments. If you are watching television or reading a novel, do so with a heart open to the possibility of knowing God through things which may not appear to be all that 'spiritual'.

Saint Benedict
21 March

Reading

It is written, 'Distribution was made to each as he had need.' By this we do not say that favouritism should be shown to persons, far from it, but that infirmities should be allowed for. If someone needs less he should thank God and not be upset; if another needs more he should be humble about his weakness, and not feel important on account of the consideration shown him, and thus all members will be at peace. Above all the bad habit of grumbling must not make its appearance in any word or gesture for any reason whatever. If anyone is found guilty of this let him pay a heavy penalty

The Rule of Saint Benedict, Chapter 34.

Meditation

Saint Benedict is revered as the father of western monasticism and is particularly remembered for his spirit of tolerance and compassion towards the monks in his charge. The Rule which he devised for his community is always fair and balanced in its outlook, taking full account of human weakness, and giving the brethren ample opportunity for the exercising of patience and tolerance towards one another. Saint Benedict exhorts the abbot of a monastery to be 'merciful, ever preferring mercy to justice. Even in his corrections, let him act with prudence. Let him remember that the bruised reed must not be broken, let him strive rather to be loved than feared.' A great deal of what he wrote applies as much to people leading busy lives in the modern world as it does to members of religious orders.

Authority calls for trust and respect from those who are to be obedient, but trust and respect must be earned. The position of authority, whether it is that of a monastic or a member of a family, or the senior member of any community, exists for the benefit of the community as a whole. This would be a good time to re-evaluate our own attitudes to those in authority over us, including the civil authorities and governments. No matter what your personal feelings are for those in authority try to hold the feelings and the people in your heart before Christ, desiring the best for them and that if necessary they be better equipped to fulfil their responsibilities. If they are people for whom you have great respect and affection, give thanks for them.

Action

Try having a day which is completely free from grumbling 'in any word or gesture for any reason whatever'.

The Annunciation to The Blessed Virgin Mary
Lady Day, 25 March

Reading

Behold, I am the handmaid of the Lord; let it be to me according to your word (Luke 1:38).

Meditation

This feast, which is full of mystery and promise, comes in the middle of Lent to cheer us on. Christ, the promised one whom we are pressing on to know, runs forward to meet us when we have only half completed the journey. He longs for union with us. All that remains for us to do is to reciprocate this longing. Mary's acceptance at the moment of the Incarnation is the beginning of a universal and eternal reorientation of creation, which is repeated and reaffirmed in our own acceptance of the Christ-child among us and in our world.

The world will be changed by those who accept, who have learned to be still and encounter God, rather than by those who rush on, intent on the business of 'doing' and of achieving results. Mary's 'let it be done to me' had nothing to do with achieving. Christ himself did not set out to achieve, but to redeem failure by obedience, by allowing himself to fail in the eyes of the world, so that the world might witness the transformation of failure into triumph. Failure and every kind of death are conquered through our loving obedience to his call in the silence of our hearts.

Action

Tomorrow is Mothering Sunday when, through Mary, and the Church, often thought of as 'Mother Church', we honour our mothers. In the last century it was also customary for young men and women in domestic service to be allowed home to visit their mothers. They would take with them a Simnel cake, named after Simon and Nelly, a brother and sister who made a cake to take to their mother but disagreed as to whether it should be baked or boiled. In the end, they baked one half and boiled the other and stuck the two together, dividing them with a layer of marzipan.

If you have children who are old enough to cook, here is a recipe for Simnel cake which they can prepare in time for tomorrow:

INGREDIENTS

550g (1¼lb) mixed dried fruit. You can include apricots which give the cake a heavier and richer consistency.
75g (3oz) mixed candied peel, chopped
225g (8oz) plain flour
A pinch of salt
1 level tsp each of ground cinnamon and nutmeg
175g (6oz) butter or margarine
175g (6oz) castor sugar
3 eggs, beaten. If the eggs are small, add an extra one.
Milk to mix
Apricot jam or marmalade to use under the almond paste
Glacé icing (optional)

Marzipan is the distinguishing feature of this cake and its most crucial ingredient. Shop-bought marzipan cannot possibly compare with the real thing, so here is a recipe for real marzipan which takes very little time and has a distinctive flavour of its own. It is well worth the effort.

For the marzipan
   450g (1lb) ground almonds
   225g (½lb) finely sieved icing sugar
   225g (½lb) castor sugar
   2 small eggs (beat the eggs together with a fork before adding them and only add them a little at a time to prevent the mixture becoming too wet and sticky. Only use as much egg as you need to get a good stiff consistency.)
   Juice of ½ a lemon
   1 tbsp of sherry or rum
   1 tbsp of orange flower water (available at a chemist)
   A few drops of almond essence

Mix the castor sugar, icing sugar and the almonds thoroughly together in a bowl. Pour in the lightly beaten eggs and the other liquids and work to a paste.

Line a 7-inch cake tin. Divide the almond paste into two. Take one portion and roll it out to a round the size of the cake tin.

Using the remaining ingredients (clean the fruit if necessary), mix the prepared currants, sultanas and peel with the flour, salt and spices. Cream the butter and sugar until pale and fluffy. Add the eggs a little at a time, beating well after each addition. Fold in half the flour and fruit, using a tablespoon, then fold in the rest. Put half of the mixture into the prepared tin, smooth and cover with the round of almond paste. Put the remaining cake mixture on top. Bake in the centre of the oven for about 1 hour. Lower the heat to cool (150°C, 300°F, mark 2). If you are using an Aga, you can slide in the metal shelf above the cake at this point, or cover the cake with foil, but whatever you do, keep an eye on it to see that it doesn't burn. Bake for 3 hours until the cake is golden-brown, firm to the touch and responds positively to the skewer test. (Insert a skewer into the centre of the cake. If there is no cake mixture sticking to it when you take it out, the cake should be done.)

Take the other half of the marzipan mixture and roll it out to a round the size of the tin. You can also make this cake as an Easter cake, in which case you need to have divided the almond paste into three, using the last third to make eleven balls (for the eleven apostles left after Judas had gone) to place in a circle on top of the cake. Brush the top of the cake with the marmalade or jam and place the second layer of marzipan on top. Decorate with a thin layer of glacé icing, made by mixing 3 tablespoons of icing sugar with enough lemon juice to make it possible for the mixture to coat the back of a spoon.

Fourth Sunday in Lent
Mothering Sunday

Reading

*After this Jesus went to the other side of the Sea of Galilee,
which is the Sea of Tiberias. And a multitude followed him,
because they saw the signs which he did on those who were
diseased. Jesus went up on the mountain, and there sat down with
his disciples.*

*Now the Passover, the feast of the Jews, was at hand. Lifting
up his eyes then, and seeing that a multitude was coming to him,
Jesus said to Philip, 'How are we to buy bread, so that these
people may eat?' This he said to test him, for he himself knew
what he would do. Philip answered him, 'Two hundred denarii
would not buy enough bread for each of them to get a little.' One
of his disciples, Andrew, Simon Peter's brother, said to him,
'There is a lad here who has five barley loaves and two fish; but
what are they among so many?' Jesus said, 'Make the people sit
down.' Now there was much grass in the place; so the men sat
down, in number about five thousand. Jesus then took the loaves,
and when he had given thanks, he distributed them to those who
were seated; so also the fish, as much as they wanted. And when
they had eaten their fill, he told his disciples, 'Gather up the
fragments left over, that nothing may be lost.' So they gathered
them up and filled twelve baskets with fragments from the five
barley loaves, left by those who had eaten. When the people saw
the sign which he had done, they said, 'This is indeed the prophet
who is to come into the world!' (John 6:1–14).*

Meditation

Try to experience this scene which must have been one of the most spectacular in the whole of Jesus's ministry. Five thousand people (enough to fill a football stadium) leave their houses and jobs one day in order to hear him speak. They have made no preparations. They simply down tools and go. Go with them as they prepare to cross the Sea of Galilee in a flotilla of little boats. Experience the warm spring sunshine and the mad joy of it all. Sit with the people on the grassy hill and look into the eyes of Jesus as he asks Philip, perhaps with a twinkle in his eye, how they are to be fed. Put yourself in Philip's place. Experience what he felt and answer for him.

These people were not driven by mere curiosity – the desire to see a few clever tricks – but by a deep need for God of which they may not have been conscious, but for which they instinctively sought satisfaction. Do we recognise our own need? Do we seek to satisfy it?

Action

Today is also known as refreshment Sunday, the day when we can loosen our belts as far as Lenten observances are concerned.

If it is a fine day, go for a picnic. If not, here is Martha Rose Shulman's recipe for barley bannocks (the nearest I could get to barley loaves) which you can have for tea at home:

INGREDIENTS

115g (4oz) barley meal
170g (6oz) 85 per cent wholemeal flour or unbleached flour
1 tsp tartaric acid
$\frac{1}{4}$ tsp salt
30g (1oz) lard or margarine

30g (1oz) unsalted butter, softened
1 tsp bicarbonate of soda
120ml (4 fl oz) buttermilk

Sift together the barleymeal, flour, tartaric acid and salt. Rub in the lard or margarine and the butter. (This can be done in a food processor fitted with a steel blade, using the pulse action, or in a mixer.) Dissolve the bicarbonate of soda in the buttermilk and when the buttermilk begins to bubble add it to the flour mixture. Bring together into a soft, sticky dough, and pat it out on a floured work surface to ½-inch thickness. Cut the dough into two large rounds – larger than a scone, but not so large that they are difficult to handle as the dough is delicate and will fall apart easily. Place them on a hot griddle. Cook them on each side for about 8–10 minutes, until the bannocks are brown and baked through. Use a wide spatula to turn them. Cool the bannocks on a rack, or serve them hot.

Fourth Week in Lent
Monday

Reading

For behold, I create new heavens and a new earth; and the former things shall not be remembered or come into mind. But be glad and rejoice for ever in that which I create; for behold, I create Jerusalem a rejoicing, and her people a joy. I will rejoice in Jerusalem, and be glad in my people; no more shall be heard in it the sound of weeping and the cry of distress. No more shall there be in it an infant that lives but a few days, or an old man who does not fill out his days, for the child shall die a hundred years old, and the sinner a hundred years old shall be accursed (Isa. 65:17–20).

Meditation

As Christ goes forward into the heart of darkness we are left with the promise of the Resurrection and of new life in all things. As a man, Christ makes himself unknowing of the joy and the triumph which lie ahead, so that we might always rejoice, even in our darkest times.

Joy is deeper and infinitely greater than passing happiness. It is the certainty of the coming dawn at the darkest moment of the night. It is the knowledge of life quietly germinating in the apparently dead seed which is buried in the cold earth.

Soon we shall go forward with Christ into Passiontide, into what had to be for him darkness without the hope of dawn. Go with him a little of the way, experiencing the early spring, the bright sheen on the grass, new young plants emerging in the light and everywhere the promise of life. Be conscious of the life which Jesus is about to lay down, for his life, like ours, is bound up in the created world and the changing seasons.

Action

Go for a walk and experience the newness of spring in plants, reflections on water, and the sky itself.

Fourth Week in Lent
Tuesday

Reading

God is our refuge and strength,
a very present help in trouble.
Therefore we will not fear though the
earth should change,
though the mountains shake
in the heart of the sea;
though its waters roar and foam,
though the mountains tremble with
its tumult.
There is a river whose streams make
glad the city of God,
the holy habitation of the Most High.
God is in the midst of her, she shall
not be moved;
God will help her right early.
The nations rage, the kingdoms
totter;
he utters his voice, the earth melts.
The Lord of hosts is with us;
The God of Jacob is our refuge
(Ps. 46:1–7).

Meditation

Not fearing something has nothing to do with not feeling frightened. Courageous people are also afraid, or they would not be courageous. Watching the news, reading the news-papers, being a part of the world we live in, aware of the possibility of ecological holocaust or sudden outbreak of war is frightening. We live with fear and sooner or later it finds expression, usually in more violence. Our society's obsession with violence is perhaps its way of running away from the fear of ultimate annihilation by making annihilation seem like fantasy.

But God is present to all of this. We shall not be moved, which is not to say that frightening things will not happen around us, or even that we may not ourselves be the victims of violence. A person who seeks God could just as easily be murdered, or the victim of an earthquake as anyone else. The difference lies in the fact that the one whose life or whose way of thinking is centred on God exists in the context of a time which is greater than the present moment. The present mo-ment with all its suffering, on both a global and a personal scale, is part of a much greater picture or plan.

Take the time to centre in the love and steadfastness of God. Settle your mind on some image, picture or idea that speaks to you directly of impregnable strength – a lighthouse on a rock perhaps, or even the living room of your own house. Know with your heart that Christ is that strength in your life, his Spirit the force which energises and inspires you.

Action

Take time to experience God as rock and refuge in the midst of the whirlpool of modern life. If you find yourself in a stressful situation where there is the possibility for tension or conflict (waiting on a crowded platform for an overcrowded tube train, at any kind of meeting where heartfelt and conflicting views are under discussion, at a family meal or gathering where an ugly row seems imminent, to name but a few examples) try for a few seconds to take time out of the situation to centre yourself and the other people around you into the sure knowledge of the omnipotent and loving God.

This is not an exercise in opting out of reality. On the contrary, with practice it makes us more fully present to the real world and to the daily conflicts and struggles in which we must, as ordinary human beings, take part.

Fourth Week in Lent
Wednesday

Reading

*As for you, my flock, thus says the Lord God: Behold, I judge
between sheep and sheep, rams and he-goats. Is it not enough for
you to feed on the good pasture, that you must tread down with
your feet the rest of your pasture; and to drink of clear water,
that you must foul the rest with your feet? And must my sheep
eat what you have trodden with your feet, and drink what you
have fouled with your feet?*

*Therefore, thus says the Lord God to them: Behold, I, I myself
will judge between the fat sheep and the lean sheep. Because you
push with side and shoulder, and thrust at all the weak with your
horns, till you have scattered them abroad, I will save my flock,
they shall no longer be a prey; and I will judge between sheep and
sheep. And I will set up over them one shepherd ... And I, the
Lord, will be their God, and my servant David shall be prince
among them; I, the Lord, have spoken.*

(Ezek. 34:17–24).

Meditation

Greed and selfishness make us blind to the enormous wealth
which is already ours in the shape of the earth and of all the
good things which it is capable of yielding. But our feet have
long since trodden down what was good and young to the
point of destroying the irreplaceable. We have trodden holes
in the delicate web of the sky, so that the pasture which was
given to us to feed on, and even our own skins, are at risk from

the dangerous rays of the sun. The plundering of the earth and its resources, the havoc we wreak with our environment – ecocide – is the sin and scourge of the age we live in.

In the final day we shall surely be held to account for every felled tree, for every wild animal that has suffocated on a plastic bag or damaged itself on a piece of litter mindlessly dropped in the countryside, for the ravaged beauty of our seas and lakes and for the indiscriminate murder of the life they hold. For God is Lord of all creation. Is it therefore inconceivable that the vast majority of those at his right hand on that terrible day will be the creatures and plants, the planets and moons that we have desecrated and then tossed aside? Perhaps in some terrifying way which we do not understand they themselves will be the judges of those who once had dominion over them.

Action

Do a little research into some of the organisations which campaign for the protection and preservation of our environment and support them in some practical way.

Fourth Week in Lent
Thursday

Reading

And the Lord said to Moses, 'Go down; for your people, whom you brought up out of the land of Egypt, have corrupted themselves; they have turned aside quickly out of the way which I commanded them; they have made for themselves a molten calf and have worshipped it and sacrificed to it, and said, "These are your gods, O Israel, who brought you up out of the land of Egypt!" ' And the Lord said to Moses, 'I have seen this people, and behold, it is a stiff-necked people; now therefore let me alone, that my wrath may burn hot against them and I may consume them; but of you I will make a great nation.'

But Moses besought the Lord his God, and said, 'O Lord, why does thy wrath burn hot against thy people, whom thou hast brought forth out of the land of Egypt with great power and with a mighty hand? Why should the Egyptians say, "With evil intent did he bring them forth, to slay them in the mountains, and to consume them from the face of the earth?" Turn from thy fierce wrath, and repent of this evil against thy people. Remember Abraham, Isaac, and Israel, thy servants, to whom thou didst swear by thine own self, and didst say to them, "I will multiply your descendants as the stars of heaven, and all this land that I have promised I will give to your descendants, and they shall inherit it for ever." ' And the Lord repented of the evil which he thought to do to his people (Exod. 32:7–14).

Meditation

It seems strange that God should put himself in the position of 'repenting', of turning back, of reorientating himself towards us, that we might come to do the same towards him. It seems equally strange that he should allow himself to be called upon to remember his promises. But God seems to prefer waiting, rather than visiting wrath and revenge on us for our ignorance of where true fulfilment lies. He waits while people drive themselves through a lifetime of believing that fulfilment and happiness lie in material achievement or possessions, or social status, or physical beauty, or any of the secret obsessions which drive us. His anger, if it is anger as we understand it, is similar to that of the loving parent who gives an offspring something precious, at great personal cost, so that the child can benefit from it and grow closer to the parent. If the present, which is God himself in the person of Christ, is tossed aside, or trampled on, or ignored in favour of some futile pastime or obsession with work, it is easy to understand how God must feel about it.

The things we love to do in life, whether they are to do with work or relationships (spouses and children can be false gods to some) are things to enjoy fully and be thankful, remembering however that they do not belong to us. They are not the source of life, but part of the gift of life from the author of life.

Spend some time reorientating yourself and taking an objective look at your priorities. Is the life you lead correctly balanced or are there obsessive areas? Does work take precedence over relationships? Loving commitment to another person with the sacrifices and responsibilities which that entails is the beginning of a loving commitment to God.

Action

If you are married take the time to sit down with your partner and take stock of where your lives, both jointly and separately, are going. Try to create a stress-free environment for this very important conversation by making sure that the air is cleared of any previous disagreements, that children are happily occupied or asleep and, if possible, that you will not be interrupted by the phone.

If you live alone assess your own priorities and how they affect the overall direction which your life is taking, as well as what effect they have on others.

Fourth Week in Lent
Friday

Reading

After this Jesus went about in Galilee; he would not go about in Judea, because the Jews sought to kill him. Now the Jews' feast of Tabernacles was at hand. But after his brothers had gone up to the feast, then he also went up, not publicly but in private. Some of the people of Jerusalem therefore said, 'Is not this the man whom they seek to kill? And here he is, speaking openly, and they say nothing to him! Can it be that the authorities really know that this is the Christ? Yet we know where this man comes from; and when the Christ appears, no one will know where he comes from.' So Jesus proclaimed, as he taught in the temple, 'You know me, and you know where I come from? But I have not come of my own accord; he who sent me is true, and him you do not know. I know him, for I come from him, and he sent me.' So they sought to arrest him; but no one laid hands on him, because his hour had not yet come (John 7:1, 2, 10, 25–30).

Meditation

With God things are never quite as we expect them to be, probably because we do not understand his ways as they are meant to be understood. Our perception of what is good and holy is often narrow and pragmatic. The good and the holy frequently come heavily disguised, and goodness is all the more difficult to discern because our senses have been numbed by a materialist and humanist conditioning which obscures these qualities when they present themselves.

144

Perhaps one of the things which most angered those who sought Christ's life was that he was simply not what their unimaginative minds had led them to believe the Messiah ought to be. Worse still, he did not fit in with their scheme of things. He was supposed to appear dramatically out of nowhere and change the face of the earth overnight, or at least deliver them from foreign domination. Instead his glory was manifested to them in the ordinary.

Things have not changed much in two thousand years. We are still seeking the way, the truth and the life through predictable channels and in predictable places (the representatives of the institutional Church, and the various authorities who run our lives for example), but Christ is to be found anywhere and everywhere. His perfection is often mirrored in the most unlikely and yet in the most obvious people. The smallest act of courtesy, a joke or a smile which has the effect of lightening a person's day, the tiniest favour, are in themselves holy and a manifestation of the living Christ in our midst.

Action

Be open to the manifestation of Christ in the kindness of another person. It could be someone you know well maybe in a shop or at work. If you recognise the moment for what it is from your heart, your response to the person will also be a little 'epiphany'.

Fourth Week in Lent
Saturday

Reading

The first man was from the earth, a man of dust; the second man is from heaven. As was the man of dust, so are those who are of the dust; and as is the man of heaven, so are those who are of heaven. Just as we have borne the image of the man of dust, we shall also bear the image of the man of heaven. I tell you this, brethren: flesh and blood cannot inherit the kingdom of God, nor does the perishable inherit the imperishable.

Lo! I tell you a mystery. We shall not all sleep, but we shall all be changed, in a moment, in the twinkling of an eye, at the last trumpet. For the trumpet will sound, and the dead will be raised imperishable, and we shall be changed.

For this perishable nature must put on the imperishable, and this mortal nature must put on immortality. When the perishable puts on the imperishable, and the moral puts on immortality, then shall come to pass the saying that is written: 'Death is swallowed up in victory. O death, where is thy victory? O death, where is thy sting?' The sting of death is sin, and the power of sin is the law (1Cor. 15:47–56).

From the readings chosen for the Orthodox Liturgy
in commemoration of the Icon of
The Most Holy Theotokos, 'The Life-giving Spring'

Meditation

We are to be utterly transformed – refurbished. Christ is a new garment which we put on in celebration of the Spring and of new life. He is new life itself.

Everything wears out in time and all living things eventually die, but the wonder of the living Christ is not so much a matter of never experiencing physical death, as of the transformation of every kind of death into part of a process for renewal and new life. Death, in all its manifestations, is no more than a stage on a journey. The end of a holiday, the end of a love affair, the end of one's schooldays – all these minor deaths are in reality a new beginning, because Christ has given us the new garment of himself to wear in them, so that we and the situation may be transformed into something imperishable and ultimately victorious. Paul speaks of these things happening 'at the last trumpet', but they have already begun to happen in the silent and secret courage of the individual's confrontation with today's dying.

Action

Affirm our refurbishment in Christ by transforming something old and tatty into something new. Polishing brass or a much-used frying pan is an excellent way of focusing on our transformation and on the transformation of unhappy situations into something new and imperishable. You could also try restoring a piece of furniture, or stripping some old paint off a wall, or redecorating a room.

To give extra lustre to a varnished or highly polished piece of furniture:

Mix 1 part of boiled linseed oil with 1 part of turpentine. Apply the mixture with a soft cloth and wipe off with a dry one. Finish by polishing with a clean dry duster until you have a perfect shine.

Passion Sunday

Reading

Behold, the days are coming, says the Lord, when I will make a new covenant with the house of Israel and the house of Judah, not like the covenant which I made with their fathers when I took them by the hand to bring them out of the land of Egypt, my covenant which they broke, though I was their husband, says the Lord.

But this is the covenant which I will make with the house of Israel after those days, says the Lord: I will put my law within them, and I will write it upon their hearts; and I will be their God, and they shall be my people. And no longer shall each man teach his neighbour and each his brother, saying, 'Know the Lord,' for they shall all know me, from the least of them to the greatest, says the Lord; for I will forgive their iniquity, and I will remember their sin no more. (Jer. 31:31–4).

Meditation

This is the beginning of Passion Week and a prelude to Holy Week itself which begins next Sunday. It is a good time to review whatever has come out of Lent and to give thanks for it, even if it was painful. There is no growth without a degree of discomfort and Lent is a time of growth and renewal.

Discerning truth in the written or spoken word, or in music or painting, means that the truth is recognised as something we know already, with which we are very familiar but have not been able to articulate. Reading a book, painting or looking at a picture (they are complementary activities), listening to music, are all part of the process of seeking and of recognising the truth which we already know because it already dwells in us. It is the law written on our hearts. These are all ways of seeking God, the truth whom we recognise and know and who is continually revealing himself in the ordinary business of living.

The 'law' which is written in us is God's presence, his union with us, so we encounter him everywhere, even in places or situations which seem far removed from prayer or spirituality. We come across him in flashes of inexplicable happiness, or in the moments of profound grief experienced at the injustice and suffering endured by others.

God is united to his world, even in its utmost depravity. But he is also one with us in the complexity and beauty of creation. We are united to the Creator God in our wholesome need for the plants and animals who share our existence and in our need for each other. Our union with him is ratified by the earth itself, as though our names were traced on his heart in soil and sand.

Action

Affirm the truth, God's law written in your heart, by doing something creative. Try painting or drawing. You could gather together a group of familiar objects and draw them as you feel them, rather than merely trying to represent what your eye is seeing. In fact in this exercise it is important to get right away from literal interpretation. Don't worry about the correct way to do things, simply enjoy the process of drawing or painting and unspoken truths will be revealed to you in the process. All creative work is a dialogue with truth and therefore with God himself.

Monday in Passion Week

Reading

The Lord is my shepherd, I shall not want;
he makes me lie down in green pastures.
He leads me beside still waters;
                    he restores my soul.
He leads me in paths of righteousness
                    for his name's sake.

Even though I walk through the
                    valley of the shadow of death,
                         I fear no evil;
for thou art with me;
                    thy rod and thy staff,
                    they comfort me.

Thou preparest a table before me
                    in the presence of my enemies;
thou anointest my head with oil,
                    my cup overflows.
Surely goodness and mercy shall follow me
                    all the days of my life;
and I shall dwell in the house of the Lord for ever
                                        (Ps. 23).

Meditation

There is no place of darkness that Christ has not visited.
The walk to Calvary is his own journeying into and

through the most painful moment of our lives as individuals. The weight of the Cross is the weight of the world's suffering since the beginning of time. Therefore we are not alone and though we walk through the valley of the shadow of death, we are shepherded by the one who goes on before us to try out the path which lies ahead, as a shepherd might make sure that a bridge is safe for the flock to cross.

Even in times of darkness we are overwhelmed with blessings, the blessing of the oil of gladness which keeps the heart supple to love and to continue to rejoice in life. Gladness lies in wait for us in unlikely times and places.

When depression wraps us in itself like a winding sheet about a corpse and the door of the tomb seems closed for ever, it is important to try with every bit of emotional strength that we have left to allow the heart and the intelligence, which have been anointed with the oil of gladness, to see and be receptive to the presence of Christ in the heart of our darkness.

Action

If you suffer from depression try holding something familiar which you associate with moments of feeling comforted. I have done this particular exercise using a Russian rosary. In holding it I am comforted by its familiar texture and I feel the strength of the Jesus Prayer flowing from it through my hand and arm to my heart. I don't actually say the prayer at times like this. I just hold the rosary. Any object will do that is familiar and comforting. A letter from a friend, a Bible or a favourite book, even a favourite cooking utensil. Nothing is ridiculous if it is an effective reminder of Christ's presence in our pain.

Also, devote as much energy as possible to being genuinely thankful for the people and things which you love.

If you know of someone else who is depressed, be a good shepherd to them, not by chivvying and harrying them into 'cheering up', but by being present to their darkness in silence and compassion.

Tuesday in Passion Week

Reading

The Lord God has given me the tongue of a teacher, that I may know how to sustain the weary with a word. Morning by morning he wakens – wakens my ear to listen as those who are taught. The Lord God has opened my ear, and I was not rebellious, I did not turn backward. I gave my back to those who struck me, and my cheeks to those who pulled out the beard; I did not hide my face from insult and spitting. The Lord God helps me; therefore I have not been disgraced; therefore I have set my face like flint, and I know that I shall not be put to shame; he who vindicates me is near. Who will contend with me? Let us stand up together. Who are my adversaries? Let them confront me. It is the Lord God who helps me; who will declare me guilty? All of them will wear out like a garment; the moth will eat them up. (Isa. 50:4–9 NRSV).

Meditation

Our kinship with Christ entitles us to his Holy Spirit. God's spirit of inspiration, intelligence and creativity is his legacy to us. The Holy Spirit continually invites us to understand God in new ways and inspires us to new language and styles of worship. Morning by morning we are wakened to that invitation, if only we will take the time to listen. It fires and motivates our every thought and action. Nothing is possible without the Spirit.

Think for a moment how easy it is to embark on a project, full of energy and enthusiasm, only to run aground after a few days or a few hours. Inspiration does not come out of the blue, neither does it depend on mood or luck. It has to be awaited and invited with active and attentive energy. It has to be allowed and obeyed. We go with God's Creator Spirit in anything we undertake, as a boat sails with the tide or current. To do things in one's own way and for one's own ends is to sail against the current and to obstruct the action of God's divine inspiration. We therefore surrender to that movement in us and through us, that we may sustain those that are weary and contend with our adversaries.

If you are involved in a project that has gone stale, or if you are undecided about a course of action, try to allow for God's Holy Spirit to enter into it. Abandon, at least for the moment, your personal views regarding its ultimate shape or outcome. Allow it to speak to you.

You can also use this prayer of Saint Ignatius to help center all of your intentions and desires into the intention and desire of God:

Take, Lord, and receive all my liberty, my memory, my understanding, and my entire will – all that I have and call my own. You have given it all to me. To you, Lord, I return it. Everything is yours; do with it what you will. Give me only your love and your grace. That is enough for me.

Action

If possible, take a day off from a project in which you are currently engaged so as to recharge your batteries and acquire a more objective outlook on it. If the idea of stopping makes you feel tense and worried about meeting a deadline or just getting the job done, organise the day in such a way as to be able to take at least an hour for some completely different creative activity. For example, if you are a painter, try writing a poem or a short piece of descriptive or journalist prose. If your project is more practical try painting or music. Treat the time as 'play'. Relax and allow yourself to enjoy it.

Wednesday in Passion Week

Reading

Then the righteous will stand with great confidence in the presence of those who have oppressed them and those who make light of their labours. When the unrighteous see them, they will be shaken with dreadful fear, and they will be amazed at the unexpected salvation of the righteous. They will speak to one another in repentance, and in anguish of spirit they will groan, and say, 'These are persons whom we once held in derision and made a byword of reproach – fools that we were! We thought that their lives were madness and that their end was without honour. Why have they been numbered among the children of God? And why is their lot among the saints? So it was we who strayed from the way of truth, and the light of righteousness did not shine on us, and the sun did not rise upon us. We took our fill of the paths of lawlessness and destruction, and we journeyed through trackless deserts, but the way of the Lord we have not known. What has our arrogance profited us? And what good has our boasted wealth brought us?' (Wisd. 5:1–8).

Meditation

This is not an excuse to feel smug or self-satisfied, or to look down on those whose ethics and opinions do not tally with our own. Neither is it an invitation to try to 'convert' people. It is, however, a message of reassurance and of hope for those who may be feeling that persevering in prayer and in a closer walk with God, at the cost of being thought 'religious' is all rather a waste of time. No obvious good seems to come of it.

It might be worth spending a minute or two remembering or imagining what life would feel like without regular times of prayer, what it feels like to be too busy or preoccupied for God. It is easy to imagine, briefly, that we would be leading an unrestrained and totally free existence. We could do all sorts of things, say all sorts of things, think all sorts of thoughts and indulge all sorts of whims which at the moment we feel gently constrained from doing. But if the constraints were removed, we would simply wander in circles and discover sooner or later that what we took to be a wide open space of independence and freedom was in fact a 'trackless waste'. We would panic inwardly because the light of Christ would not be there to guide us home. This is what the world has to offer and from which so many are driven to seek oblivion in work, in frenetic activity to fill out their loneliness, in alchohol, and in every kind of addiction.

Spend some time holding the world's pain and loneliness before Christ without in any way passing judgment on those who suffer, but feeling for them as loved members of your own family. This may work better for one or two people personally known to you, but in any case let no trace of superiority creep into this time with them. Forget who you are and get into their situation, seeing and feeling as they do.

Action

Consider the possibility of giving some time to working for one of the charities which seek to alleviate the suffering of the destitute or of drug addicts and alcoholics.

Thursday in Passion Week

Reading

For a brief moment I forsook you, but with great compassion I will gather you. In overflowing wrath for a moment I hid my face from you, but with everlasting love I will have compassion on you, says the Lord, your Redeemer. For this is like the days of Noah to me: as I swore that the waters of Noah should no more go over the earth, so I have sworn that I will not be angry with you and will not rebuke you. For the mountains may depart and the hills be removed, but my steadfast love shall not depart from you, and my covenant of peace shall not be removed, says the Lord, who has compassion on you (Isa. 54:7–10).

Meditation

Imagine or remember what it was like to be really angry with a child. Remember or imagine what you felt at the time, how patient you had been until then, how you were feeling that day. Perhaps you were tired or worried about something. The child in question had committed the same offence for the hundredth time and this was the last straw.

Usually we lose our temper with our children because they test our patience to the limit. Ask yourself if you ever really stopped loving the child, even though in the heat of the moment you may not have felt all that loving.

God is a parent to us and also a spouse and lover, but infinitely more patient, infinitely fairer and more generous towards us than we are towards our own children, wanting more than anything the reciprocation of his love for us and our happiness and well-being in the freedom he gives us. Imagine therefore his feelings as a loving parent, as the spouse of his people at the state of the world and at the indifference of individuals towards him.

Action

Experience parental love – even if you don't have children of your own – by taking a younger member of your family, or any child known to you, for a treat.

Friday in Passion Week

Reading

I lift up my eyes to the hills.
            From whence does my help come?
My help comes from the Lord,
            who made heaven and earth.

He will not let your foot be moved,
            he who keeps you will not slumber.
Behold, he who keeps Israel
            will neither slumber nor sleep.

The Lord is your keeper;
            the Lord is your shade on your right hand.
The sun shall not smite you by day,
            nor the moon by night.

The Lord will keep you from all evil;
            he will keep your life.
your going out and your coming in
from this time forth and for evermore (Ps. 121).

Meditation

It is never easy to think beautiful thoughts in the midst of
depression, anxiety or sickness. Sometimes one's own inner
state of darkness is so impenetrable and so all-consuming that

one feels that God has in some way departed – like a small child must feel whose mother has left the room.

Thinking scientifically can help to ground this kind of desolation in reality. An awareness of the order and harmony of the created world helps to rationalise our feelings and earths us in the complex order of the life which sustains us.

If I look out of my window I see a paddock with one or two old fruit trees in it, as well as two magnificent beeches and a number of evergreens and conifers where the woods which are outside my house begin to advance on the field. In May the field is full of bluebells, wild campion and the last of the wild daffodils. All is vibrant with the year's new colour. Its complexity is fixed and it thrives and depends for its continued growth on the seasons and on my husband's patient mowing. Somehow, I too, am part of this mutually dependent order. I am kept in its shade and it seems that even my going out and my coming in are linked to the growth of the grass and to the season's fresh leaves. All of this growth and fruitfulness, with all the promise and potential, enters my sad and sullen heart. I am a part of the universe, at one with it. I am kept safe and held in place by the Lord who made heaven and earth.

Extend these thoughts to a place which you love. Feel in your heart the good and healing memories which it brings. Draw into these memories the people, living or dead, with whom you associate the place. Continue to love them and if they are no longer alive, give thanks for them and wish them in the Father's house.

Action

Whether or not you are feeling depressed, take time to look out of a window with a view which is in any way familiar or pleasing. You don't have to live in the country. We can sense our oneness with creation and with the rest of humanity by contemplating a landscape of roofs and television aerials, or a busy street. The important thing is to realise our bond with the created world and with one another, all of which is held with great tenderness as a single and composite whole by the Maker of all things visible and invisible.

Saturday in Passion Week

Reading

Jesus answered them, 'Destroy this temple, and in three days I will raise it up.' The Jews then said, 'This temple has been under construction for forty-six years, and will you raise it up in three days?' But he was speaking of the temple of his body. After he was raised from the dead, his disciples remembered that he had said this; and they believed the scripture and word that Jesus had spoken.

When he was in Jerusalem during the Passover festival, many believed in his name because they saw the signs that he was doing. But Jesus on his part would not entrust himself to them, because he knew all people and needed no one to testify about anyone; for he himself knew what was in everyone (John 2:19–end NRSV).

Meditation

Jesus knew the fickleness of human nature. He knew it in the most profound sense, without being fickle or false himself, and yet at the same time with the knowledge that can only come from experience. He trusted himself to no one and so experienced intense loneliness.

The destruction of the temple of which he speaks was the annihilation of his inner self, and of his dreams, as well as of his physical body. It was the ultimate disillusion. There is a kind of dying which is not purely physical but which involves the shattering of illusions and dreams by circumstances or by other people. It also involves not belonging to any place or group in particular, not qualifying as a something or a someone.

In the times in which we live this kind of death can be the loneliest of all, but the Resurrection in which we share as brothers and sisters of Christ means that we belong with him in our Father's house. Christ has gone ahead of us in the pain and mess of the human predicament to mend what is broken and to raise up what is fallen and far from perfection in ourselves and in our society.

If you have experienced the shattering of your own dreams, take heart in knowing that Christ himself is present to your pain.

This is the beginning of Holy Week when the Church's liturgy for each day of the week follows as closely as possible the events of Christ's Passion, culminating with the Resurrection on Easter Sunday.

Action

Admit your own brokenness and, if you have suffered disappointments, bring empathy and real understanding to someone known to you who is in a similar position.

Palm Sunday

Reading

And the soldiers led him away inside the palace (that is, the praetorium); and they called together the whole battalion. And they clothed him in a purple cloak, and plaiting a crown of thorns they put it on him. And they began to salute him, 'Hail, King of the Jews!' And they struck his head with a reed, and spat upon him, and they knelt down in homage to him. And when they had mocked him, they stripped him of the purple cloak, and put his own clothes on him. And they led him out to crucify him (Mark 15:16–21).

Meditation

Try to be present to this moment and open to experiencing what any of the people present might have been feeling in that barracks. A battalion comprised some forty soldiers who made sport of their victims. There were usually three prisoners condemned to scourging at any one time and scourging was itself a softening-up process prior to crucifixion, to ensure, among other things, that the victims did not take too long to die. The three drew lots to see who would be punished first and the one who was chosen was called the King. Some were driven insane by what was inflicted on them.

Imagine the mood of the soldiers, drunk, raucous and licensed to indulge in both mental and physical sadism. Feel for Christ who in a mysterious way both knew and did not know who they were, their backgrounds, their families, their fears and hopes. Experience for a second his vulnerability towards them – his allowing of love for them.

Next time you hear a child laugh or are made aware of the special quality of sunlight on a late summer's afternoon, or feel an inexplicable surge of happiness, remember that these are just some of the gifts which have been bought and paid for by Christ's Passion. We and the whole of creation were bought with a price. He holds in himself our pain and our loss, and our futility and failure are made good in him. In his humiliation and defeat we are made new. By his stripes we are healed.

Action

There will not always be a practical action during Holy Week, so let whatever happens in the course of the meditations colour your outlook for the entire day.

Monday in Holy Week

Reading

Now when Jesus was at Bethany in the house of Simon the leper, a woman came up to him with an alabaster flask of very expensive ointment, and she poured it on his head, as he sat at table. But when the disciples saw it, they were indignant, saying, 'Why this waste? For this ointment might have been sold for a large sum, and given to the poor.' But Jesus, aware of this, said to them, 'Why do you trouble the woman? For she has done a beautiful thing to me. For you always have the poor with you, but you will not always have me. In pouring this ointment on my body she has done it to prepare me for burial. Truly, I say to you, wherever this gospel is preached in the whole world, what she has done will be told in memory of her' (Matt. 26:6–13).

Meditation

Modern worship often seems to reflect modern life. It lacks the beauty which comes of reverence. If we loved and worshipped like this woman, with greater abandon and fewer fears of the cost and the consequences of loving, we should transfigure and transform our world and our day-to-day existence. For she transfigured the moment of Christ's arrival at a party into a manifestation, an epiphany of the Saviour, by the generosity and reverence of her action.

Life and worship should be inextricably bound up in each other. Christ is revealed as Saviour through us to the world and to those whom we anoint with love. Our worship, which is made beautiful by the sort of people we are, is presented to him as a living sacrifice, made holy by the gift of himself dwelling in us.

Try to picture yourself in this situation as one of the guests, or as the woman herself and experience in your own heart what she felt. What do you feel when your action is justified?

Action

Anoint someone in your household or place of work with a caring action performed especially for them. You could put flowers in a bedroom, mend someone's favourite jeans or repair a loved piece of china, or a child's toy or bicycle. Or you could just make a beautiful thing, purely for the sake of making it and as a means of loving and worshipping God, in the way the woman in the story, believed to be Mary Magdalen, loves and worships Christ.

There was a time when visitors to a house were sprinkled with rose water – a form of anointing. You may not want to anoint people in this way as they step through the door, but here is a recipe for rose water which you can bottle and give to them as a present instead:

INGREDIENTS
400ml (16 fl oz) distilled water
50ml (2 fl oz) vodka
10 drops of rose oil
½ cup fresh, dark red rose petals

Pour the distilled water into a mixing bottle which has been thoroughly cleansed.

Add the vodka. (Don't use rubbing alcohol as it has a scent of its own which vies with that of the roses.)

Mix in the rose petals so that they are thoroughly wet, then add the oil.

Let the mixture stand in a covered bottle in a cool, dark place for one week to allow the scent to age.

Rose petals do not keep very well, even in alcohol, so it is best to remove them before transferring the mixture to a small glass bottle.

Tuesday in Holy Week

Reading

And he came out, and went, as was his custom, to the Mount of Olives; and the disciples followed him. And when he reached the place he said to them, 'Pray that you may not enter into temptation.' And he withdrew from them about a stone's throw, and knelt down and prayed, 'Father, if thou art willing, remove this cup from me; nevertheless not my will, but thine, be done.' And there appeared to him an angel from heaven, strengthening him. And being in an agony he prayed more earnestly; and his sweat became like great drops of blood falling down upon the ground. And when he rose from prayer, he came to the disciples and found them sleeping for sorrow, and he said to them, 'Why do you sleep? Rise and pray that you may not enter into temptation' (Luke 22:39–47).

Meditation

Try to experience this situation first as Christ experienced it and then as one of the disciples. Be open, relaxed and centred from the heart in a desire to meet Christ in the garden, or in some modern equivalent setting if you find it easier. Allow God's spirit to take you through some of the emotions that Jesus must have experienced as a man – the fear, the loneliness, the near despair – and let your own emotions and feelings make a dialogue with his. Then, if you like, place yourself alongside the disciples and experience what they felt – the mental and physical exhaustion, the confusion and doubt, perhaps. Note your own feelings and response on being awoken and told to watch and pray and to guard against temptation.

You can do this meditation in two stages, separating them with an interval of a few hours but if you find that one particular aspect of it speaks to you, then stay with it or repeat it later in the day.

Action

It is a good idea to write down anything that happens in this kind of prayer. Later on you will have something to go back to, as well as evidence that it really did happen. If you are keeping a journal make full use of it this week.

Wednesday in Holy Week

Reading

Then the whole company of them arose, and brought him before Pilate. And they began to accuse him, saying, 'We found this man perverting our nation, and forbidding us to give tribute to Caesar, and saying that he himself is Christ a king.' And Pilate asked him, 'Are you the King of the Jews?' And he answered him, 'You have said so.' And Pilate said to the chief priests and the multitudes, 'I find no crime in this man.' But they were urgent, saying, 'He stirs up the people, teaching throughout all Judea, from Galilee even to this place.'

When Pilate heard this, he asked whether the man was a Galilean. And when he learned that he belonged to Herod's jurisdiction, he sent him over to Herod, who was himself in Jerusalem at that time. When Herod saw Jesus, he was very glad, for he had long desired to see him, because he had heard about him, and he was hoping to see some sign done by him. So he questioned him at some length; but he made no answer. The chief priests and the scribes stood by, vehemently accusing him. And Herod with his soldiers treated him with contempt and mocked him; then, arraying him in gorgeous apparel, he sent him back to Pilate. And Herod and Pilate became friends with each other that very day, for before this they had been at enmity with each other (Luke 23:1–12).

Meditation

Be in the situation. Understand it as much as possible from the heart and understand how even at the heart of darkness Christ brings forth good. Two men who had long been at enmity with each other were now friends. Remember and understand from the heart what friendship really means and so understand the implication of this moment of healing. In the midst of conflict and suffering Christ makes good and whole, as he did when he healed the ear of the high priest's servant which was cut off by Peter earlier on in the garden.

At the same time, take with you into this situation all victims of torture and those who suffer because of perverted justice. If you have painful memories of your own, when you were treated unjustly, own them fully, no matter how insignificant they may seem in comparison to those suffered by Jesus. No suffering is ever insignificant. Go back in memory to the times when you suffered humiliation and allow Christ to stand beside you in that context.

Maundy Thursday

Reading

Now before the feast of the Passover, when Jesus knew that his hour had come to depart out of this world to the Father, having loved his own who were in the world, he loved them to the end. And during supper, when the devil had already put it into the heart of Judas Iscariot, Simon's son, to betray him, Jesus, knowing that the Father had given all things into his hands, and that he had come from God and was going to God, rose from supper, laid aside his garments, and girded himself with a towel. Then he poured water into a basin, and began to wash the disciples' feet, and to wipe them with the towel with which he was girded. He came to Simon Peter; and Peter said to him, 'Lord, do you wash my feet?' Jesus answered him, 'What I am doing you do not know now, but afterward you will understand.' Peter said to him, 'You shall never wash my feet.' Jesus answered him, 'If I do not wash you, you have no part in me.' Simon Peter said to him, 'Lord, not my feet only but also my hands and my head!' Jesus said to him, 'He who has bathed does not need to wash, except for his feet, but he is clean all over; and you are clean, but not every one of you.' For he knew who was to betray him; that was why he said, 'You are not all clean.'

When he had washed their feet, and taken his garments, and resumed his place, he said to them, 'Do you know what I have done to you? You call me Teacher and Lord; and you are right, for so I am. If I then, your Lord and Teacher, have washed your feet, you also ought to wash one another's feet. For I have given you an example, that you also should do as I have done to you.' (John 13:1–15).

Meditation

Most people who have the responsibility of caring for a family or a community know what real service is about. It involves first of all setting aside one's garments; in other words, the garments of one's image and of one's personal priorities, in order for others to grow and become fully what they were intended to be. Parents, teachers, politicians and leaders of any sort of community from a monastery to the shop floor of a factory, have the responsibility of serving others in nurturing them to a state of consummate wholeness. Nurturing others in serving them is the most profoundly rewarding occupation that life has to offer, so it is not surprising that Jesus instructed his disciples to do to each other as he was doing to them.

Humility in the service of others has nothing to do with grovelling, self-abasement, and the denial of our own potential. We are called to serve as full and free individuals, with the humility and dignity of Christ which come from having first accepted and forgiven ourselves. Only then may we set aside our own needs, to grasp the needs of another. I employ my 'self', whom I have learned to love and forgive, as a free and creative gesture in the making and building up of someone else.

Our relationship with Christ rests like Peter's on our continual allowing of his washing of our feet. It rests on his being allowed to serve us in the cleansing and healing of those hidden parts of our personality which are most in need of rest and refreshment. Let us not create obstructions for him with the inner garments of 'public face' or 'private image', for in allowing the worst of ourselves to be washed, the whole is made clean.

Action

Try having a day without some article of image-protective clothing. You could have a day without wearing makeup, or you could take a bus to work or walk, instead of going by car or taxi. You could give someone else your seat on the train. If you have a particular côterie at work with whom you normally eat lunch, try seeking out someone who has few friends and who might value your company.

If you have young children, take special care of their bodies at bathtime tonight. Cherish them, that in time they may learn to accept themselves as they are.

Passover

Reading

*Then Moses called all the elders of Israel, and said to them,
'Select lambs for yourselves according to your families, and kill
the passover lamb. Take a bunch of hyssop and dip it in the blood
which is in the basin, and touch the lintel and the two doorposts
with the blood which is in the basin; and none of you shall go out
of the door of his house until the morning. For the Lord will pass
through to slay the Egyptians; and when he sees the blood on the
lintel and on the two doorposts, the Lord will pass over the door,
and will not allow the destroyer to enter your houses to slay you.
You shall observe this rite as an ordinance for you and for your
sons for ever.'* (Exod. 12:21–4).

From the public readings chosen for Passover

Meditation

The Jewish festival of Passover lasts for eight days. It coincides
with the Spring and is partly an agricultural festival, coincid-
ing with the ripening of the winter grain. The Hebrew name
for Passover is *Pesach* meaning to pass over, and the feast is
kept in commemoration and thanksgiving for the deliverance
of the Jewish people from the first of the plagues which were
inflicted on Pharoah for refusing to allow them to leave Egypt.
All of the first-born of Egypt, including livestock, were smitten
with the plague, but the angel of death was commanded by
God to pass over and spare the houses of the Israelites. The
angel would recognise their houses because the door posts and

lintels were to be smeared with the blood of the passover lamb.

The feast is also known as the Feast of Unleavened Bread. When the time finally came for their departure from the country which had enslaved them, the Jewish people were in such a hurry to leave that they did not have time to wait for the bread to rise before it was baked, so they took with them flat loaves, known as *matzoth* which had been made without yeast. Passover is still commemorated as the Festival of Freedom and related to the universal fight against every kind of slavery and oppression.

The last supper which Jesus ate with his disciples was a *Seder*. It is the ritual Passover meal which is celebrated in the home, as opposed to the synagogue. The bread which he broke was the new covenant, the new promise of deliverance for the whole human race from the consequences of the mess, on whatever scale, which we have made of our individual lives and of the course of history. It was his body, broken down and given over for the whole of humanity. The cup was the ritual cup of wine passed around the family table at a *Seder*, now become the blood of the sacrifice of himself in which the Covenant of our salvation, our kinship with him, is sealed.

Use this time to pray for greater understanding between Christians and Jews. Understand in your own way the significance of the Cross as the New Covenant, or pact, between God and all people and be thankful for the Jewish people who were chosen by God to bring his Messiah into the world. Desire peace and justice for all who live in the Holy Land.

Action

Passover is a good time to remember and be grateful for our Jewish antecedents. Celebrating the Passover at home, or in the wider context of the parish, affirms Christianity's historical roots in the Jewish tradition. It also helps to make more sense of our own Eucharistic liturgy.

Among the foods eaten at a *Seder* are those which symbolise various aspects of the deliverance of the Jewish people from Egypt. If you are planning to have a *Seder* of your own, you will need to place the following things at the head of the table: 3 whole *matzohs* on a dish covered with a napkin, a roasted egg, a roasted meatbone, *charoses*, bitter herbs (horseradish sauce is substituted for these), a dish of salt water, and parsley. In addition to these, 4 cups of wine are drunk at specified points during the service.

The *matzohs* represent the unleavened bread eaten by the Jews as they were fleeing from Pharoah. It is also called the 'bread of affliction'. The bitter herbs, or horseradish also symbolise affliction. The meatbone is all that is left of the Paschal lamb which was traditionally sacrificed at this time. The roasted egg symbolises the freewill offering which was brought to the temple in place of the lamb. The *charoses*, along with the *matzohs*, represent the bricks which the Israelites were obliged to make for Pharoah, the *charoses* being the mortar into which the 'bricks' are dipped.

Here is a recipe for *charoses* which is used as a dip with the *matzohs*.

INGREDIENTS
    1 cup of chopped apples
    ¼ cup of chopped nuts
    1 tsp of sugar or honey
    The grated rind of ½ a lemon
    1 tsp of cinnamon
    2 tbsp of red wine (approx)

Combine these with enough wine to bind the mixture.

Good Friday

Reading

Behold the wood of the cross, on which hung the Saviour of the world.

Liturgy for the veneration of the Cross

Meditation

Stand beside Mary watching her son sigh out his life in agony. Like any mother, she would gladly take upon herself the pain and humiliation of her child – the child whose shoes she once buckled, who had his favourite food, his favourite treat, the adolescent for whom no task of hers was too menial, no sadness or concern too trivial. Keep watch with her and with John, the disciple for whom the Lord had such a special love. Accept their suffering as your own. Accept also that the indescribable suffering of Christ, experienced on so many levels, is the reality of his presence and of his claiming for himself our darkest and most secret thought or deed.

The execution of criminals takes place outside the city walls. The crosses stand on the municipal rubbish dump which is also an open sewer. It takes a certain type of person to come and watch such an event out of mere curiosity, as it takes a certain type of person to drive miles out of their way to stare in fascination at the carnage of a motorway accident. This person dwells in all of us, in one form or another.

Rats, dogs and vultures watch and wait for the pickings. The three who are being crucified experience the jeers and shouts, the rancid smell of bad wine and rotting debris as somehow moulded to the heaving earth and sky. All is joined to Christ's last cry and to all cries, all sighs, and all that is unnameable in suffering. Then black and sudden silence – no whimpering into oblivion, only an abrupt return to the emptiness of the beginning, before all worlds began.

Holy Saturday

Reading

May the light of Christ rising in glory scatter the darkness of our heart and mind.

The lighting of the Paschal Candle

Meditation

The ritual lighting of the Paschal Candle begins in a darkened room, to symbolise the darkness of the tomb, in which the glow of the New Fire is dimly reflected from outside. The taper which is used to light the candle is lit from the fire and so is the sanctuary lamp which will burn in the church throughout the coming year. When the priest has lit the Paschal Candle, more tapers are lit from it and passed around the darkened room for each of those present to light their individual candle. Suddenly the room is light, but not as with electricity, in the fraction of a second. It is more like an accelerated dawn. The fundamental condition of the room has changed, so it is not just a matter of being able to see the people and things around one, but that one somehow perceives and experiences them in a new way.

The light which issues forth from the tomb on this holy night changes our perception of life. It is the good news, told quietly, of Christ's victory over all that has gone wrong in the world, his dominion over pain and suffering and death and his harrowing of hell itself.

Action

Sometime after dark, ideally at midnight, gather the members of the household together into a darkened room and having lit a candle which can represent the Paschal Candle, let each person light a candle from the main flame. You could follow with a reading of the Creation story from Genesis 1:1–2, 4.

EASTERTIDE

Easter Sunday

Reading

Christ our passover is sacrificed for us: therefore let us keep the feast;

Not with the old leaven, nor with the leaven of malice and wickedness: but with the unleavened bread of sincerity and truth.

Christ being raised from the dead dieth no more: death hath no more dominion over him.

For in that he died, he died unto sin once: but in that he liveth, he liveth unto God.

Likewise reckon ye also yourselves to be dead indeed unto sin: but alive unto God, through Jesus Christ our Lord.

Christ is risen from the dead: and become the first fruits of them that slept.

For since by man came death: by man came also the resurrection of the dead.

For as in Adam all die: even so in Christ shall all be made alive.

Easter Anthem

Meditation

Christ is the Passover lamb who has been sacrificed for us. His Resurrection is only the beginning of a never-ending story because the living 'unto God through Jesus Christ our Lord' goes on and on in the endlessly changing and self-renewing pattern of life, in circumstances and in surprises around every corner. Easter is the Christian's Festival of Freedom because Christ our Passover has loosed us from the grave clothes of fear, prejudice and inhibition and of complexes, shortcomings and failures. All things are possible in him. Through him and in him nothing is impossible.

Easter is the time for rising from the tomb of the past in order to run with Christ, looking up and forward to a new world and to a renewal of ourselves in the fullness of his Resurrection.

Allow the triumph of Christ's Resurrection to be a source of strength, especially if you are faced with seemingly hopeless situations – illness, relationships which have gone wrong, problems and tasks which seem insurmountable. Be with the risen Christ, whatever your predicament, and know from that face-to-face encounter in sincerity and truth that all things are worked to the good for those who love him.

Action

It is customary at Easter to eat young spring lamb as a reminder of Christ's innocence and of his sacrifice of himself as the Paschal Lamb. Here is a way of cooking roast lamb which I learned from my mother:

Take a shoulder of spring lamb (the size will depend on the number of people you are feeding, but I have always found the flavour to be best when the joint is small) and with the point of a very sharp knife insert thin slivers of garlic just under the skin. You will need roughly 4 cloves of garlic for a joint weighing 5lb. Rub the underside of the joint with garlic and tuck one or two pieces of garlic into the folds of the meat. Rub the joint with soya sauce, followed by a thin coating of olive oil. Season with pepper and a plentiful quantity of fresh rosemary and thyme. Roast in the normal way.

Easter Monday

Reading

*And when the sabbath was past, Mary Magdalene, and Mary the
mother of James, and Salome, bought spices, so that they might
go and anoint him. And very early on the first day of the week they
went to the tomb when the sun had risen. And they were saying to
one another, 'Who will roll away the stone for us from the door of
the tomb?' And looking up, they saw that the stone was rolled back
– it was very large. And entering the tomb, they saw a young man
sitting on the right side, dressed in a white robe; and they were
amazed. And he said to them, 'Do not be amazed; you seek Jesus
of Nazareth, who was crucified. He has risen, he is not here; see
the place where they laid him. But go, tell his disciples and Peter
that he is going before you to Galilee; there you will see him, as he
told you.' And they went out and fled from the tomb; for trembling
and astonishment had come upon them; and they said nothing to
anyone, for they were afraid* (Mark 16:1–8).

Meditation

Some say that the young man in question was the same young
man who fled naked from the mob which came to arrest Jesus
in the garden, an angel of light in disguise. The women had
come to complete the action begun a few nights earlier at
supper in the house of Simon the leper at Bethany (see p. 167).
They were greeted instead by a messenger from heaven.
Circumstances seem woven together, but the true revelation
was yet to come.

Experience this scene for yourself. The women were not only shocked and dismayed, but confused and bewildered. Was their imagination playing tricks on them? With the events of the past few days, they were probably short of sleep. It was very early. Experience the early morning when the day lies ahead untouched. There is a kind of primal innocence about everything. Christ, in his rising from the dead, restores to us our innocence. Hear the sounds of life stirring and feel the terrible impact of his absence as you find the tomb empty. Experience from the heart the angel's message, 'He has risen'.

Action

An Easter garden is a good way to 'fix' this meditation in reality. It will also keep children busy for at least an hour.

All you need is some form of container – a bowl or large plastic box will do. An old sink works well if you are doing this outside. Fill the container with soil or sand and make a replica of the garden and the tomb using stones, moss, sticks, flowers or anything you can think of. If you use moss, remember to keep it moist.

Tuesday in Easter Week

Reading

*Open to me the gates of righteousness,
that I may enter through them
and give thanks to the Lord.*

*This is the gate of the Lord;
the righteous shall enter through it.*

*I thank thee that thou hast answered me
and hast become my salvation.
The stone which the builders rejected
has become the head of the corner.
This is the Lord's doing;
it is marvellous in our eyes.
This is the day which the Lord has made;
Let us rejoice and be glad in it*
(Ps. 118:19–24).

Meditation

This is the day. This is the time and the season for gladness, a gladness which cannot be changed or taken from us, even though at this moment we may find ourselves in a period of grief.

Gladness which springs from Christ's Resurrection is from before all things. It is the source of all things, for the Creator loved the universe into being and the 'big bang' which is the current scientific explanation for the beginning of our universe was his great shout of gladness. The Resurrection of Christ is a second 'big bang', a new creation, and all suffering is caught up in it and changed.

Pain does not go away just because it is Easter week but our pain, linked to that of the Saviour, has become the cornerstone and the means for resurrection and for a new beginning. Our broken relationships, disappointments, failures and every kind of loss are joined to the cornerstone, Christ, who is our salvation, who re-creates order and harmony out of the chaos and uncontrollable forces of suffering.

If you are going through a period of suffering try to hold the pain, hearing at the same time the shout of gladness which rings through it.

If these are good times allow yourself to be fully glad and fully grateful for your happiness.

Action

Easter eggs have their origin in the pagan rites of spring, to celebrate new life and fertility. We incorporate them into the Christian festival of Easter in celebration of the new life that is the risen Christ and to mark our gladness. Here is a basic formula for decorating Easter eggs:

Use eggs which have pale shells. If you want them plain green or red, boil them in water which has had spinach or beetroot cooked in it. For yellow eggs, try adding a teaspoonful of turmeric to the water. You can of course use food colouring. For a mottled effect, wrap the eggs in onion skin secured firmly with cotton, and if you want them patterned, try placing flower petals on the damp eggs, covering these with onion skin and securing the whole with cotton. For geometric designs, stick narrow strips of masking tape to the eggs and for each 'design' plunge them in a different coloured water. Peel off the tape at the end to reveal a pattern. Repeat this procedure several times to get a layered effect. You can also cut out miniature templates in the shape of stars or flowers which, when peeled off, will be revealed as white against a coloured background. Give a shine to the finished egg by polishing it with a little oil.

Wednesday in Easter Week

Reading

O give thanks to the Lord, call on his name,
>> *make known his deeds among the peoples!*
Sing to him, sing praises to him,
>> *tell of all his wonderful works!*
Glory in his holy name;
>> *let the hearts of those who seek the Lord rejoice!*
Seek the Lord and his strength,
>> *seek his presence continually!*
Remember the wonderful works that he has done,
>> *his miracles, and the judgments he uttered,*
O offspring of Abraham his servant,
>> *sons of Jacob, his chosen ones!*

He is the Lord our God;
>> *his judgments are in all the earth.*
He is mindful of his covenant for ever,
>> *of the word that he commanded, for a*
>> *thousand generations*

(Ps. 105: 1–8).

Meditation

Glory, seek and remember. This is the way to live prayerfully,
not with one's head in the clouds, because a person who seeks
God at all times and in all places is more in contact with the
real world than one who claims to have no interest in him.

193

Seeking God in this way involves being disposed to a glad encounter with him at unexpected moments. The French word *épanoui* means something like 'in full bloom' or radiant. Glorying in the risen Christ means having about one something of his radiance, which comes from encountering him in all sorts of places. It has nothing to do with broad smiles and cheerful faces, but more with something which wells up from within, like a spring of water discovered in some wild place.

Seeking God is a kind of cupping of the hands to receive the water which we already have within us. We still seek the water because the joy of prayer lies in going forever further into the unutterable joy which already belongs to us and which must belong to all.

We remember how the joy came to be ours in drawing into the present moment and into our daily lives the life of Christ on earth, the love of the Father in the beauty of the created world and of one another, and the life, inspiration and energy of the Holy Spirit. This is called living Eucharistically. We are not re-enacting something from the past but making it alive and relevant to the present.

Spend this time in being disposed to encounter the risen Christ and to live Eucharistically.

Action

Thank someone or show appreciation of something given or done for you, even if you've already thanked them once. Make a point of using and enjoying something which has been given to you.

Thursday in Easter Week

Reading

As they were saying this, Jesus himself stood among them. But they were startled and frightened, and supposed that they saw a spirit. And he said to them, 'Why are you troubled, and why do questionings rise in your hearts? See my hands and my feet, that it is I myself; handle me, and see; for a spirit has not flesh and bones as you see that I have.' And while they still disbelieved for joy, and wondered, he said to them, 'Have you anything here to eat?' They gave him a piece of broiled fish, and he took it and ate before them.

Then he said to them, 'These are my words which I spoke to you, while I was still with you, that everything written about me in the law of Moses and the prophets and the psalms must be fulfilled.' Then he opened their minds to understand the scriptures, and said to them, 'Thus it is written, that the Christ should suffer and on the third day rise from the dead, and that repentance and forgiveness of sins should be preached in his name to all nations, beginning from Jerusalem. You are witnesses of these things' (Luke 24:36–48).

Meditation

Anyone who has ever seen a ghost has some idea of what the apostles must have felt at this moment. But even without having seen one it is not difficult to imagine, so try putting yourself in their position. Experience the reality of the presence of Christ, what it felt like to touch him and to watch him eat. The understanding of scripture which he gives to his apostles is a kind of intellectual new dawn, a realisation of the truth. Everything falls into place once and for all. The reality and the reason for the coming of the long awaited Messiah are made plain.

In modern life a continuous face-to-face encounter with God makes us witnesses of the Resurrection. This encounter is made possible by a deliberate and conscious attitude of readiness and willingness to the appearance of Christ in our midst. It is an attitude of openness and acceptance of the reality of Christ made manifest to the individual in ways in which only that individual can apprehend him. There are no rules for encountering God – no conditions or required attributes, only a willingness to be surprised.

Action

Anchor these thoughts in something tangible, as the Saviour sought to reassure the apostles by eating in their presence.

Here is a simple way to grill fish. Red mullet is particularly good cooked liked this, but mackerel works well too.

INGREDIENTS FOR 4

6–8 red mullet, depending on the size of the fish and on your appetite
2 onions
1 lemon
1 bulb fennel
Parsley
2 cloves of garlic (optional)
Olive oil
Salt, pepper

Brush the fish lightly with olive oil. Cover them with quite thick slices of onion (about ½cm) remembering to put some inside as well. Squeeze $\frac{1}{2}$ a lemon over them, leaving the rind to cook with the fish which will accentuate the lemony flavour. Add salt, pepper and a liberal quantity of sliced fresh fennel and parsley. It is best to use bulb fennel which is fairly easy to obtain in supermarkets. Stuff the inside of the fish with the feathery leaves and the garlic. Either grill the fish, or else wrap it in foil like a parcel and bake in a fairly hot oven for about 20 minutes. Serve the fish with rice or pitta bread and a green salad, accompanied by a bottle of dry white wine. The rest of the lemon can be cut in wedges and served separately.

Friday in Easter Week

Reading

When they had finished breakfast, Jesus said to Simon Peter, 'Simon, son of John, do you love me more than these?' He said to him, 'Yes, Lord; you know that I love you.' He said to him, 'Feed my lambs.' A second time he said to him, 'Simon, son of John, do you love me?' He said to him, 'Yes, Lord; you know that I love you.' He said to him, 'Tend my sheep.' He said to him the third time, 'Simon, son of John, do you love me?' Peter was grieved because he said to him the third time, 'Do you love me?' And he said to him, 'Lord, you know everything; you know that I love you.' Jesus said to him, 'Feed my sheep' (John 21:15–17).

Meditation

The question was not, 'Are you prepared to work a fifteen-hour day for seven days a week?' It was simply a matter of love. The word 'ministry' is bandied about rather freely in certain circles. One can have a ministry for almost anything and the underlying pressure which this puts on people can get in the way of their experience of God in the context of corporate worship, as if by not having some sort of clear ministry they have somehow failed.

The question which Jesus was asking has to do with priorities. He wanted Peter to be sure that love mattered more than the work of feeding. The reason for this is that Peter's love for Christ would sustain him and enable him to be a channel of that same food and sustenance to the flock.

Going about it in a methodical and efficient manner was not what interested Jesus, and this is the mistake which Judas made when he complained that money spent on expensive ointments and perfume would have been better spent on the poor. The most conscientious ministry carried out without a consuming love for God, translated into love for the flock is ultimately ineffective.

To minister is to care for, in other words to be continually re-created in ourselves so that we can be facilitators of the process of re-creation in others. But it is only possible to care for people and places if we have first been convinced of our belonging to the God who loves us and who is become the source and the means whereby we love others. This is why the question which Jesus puts to Peter is so important and at first so baffling. The relationship with Christ comes before the personal relationship which we have with any other living thing.

All occupations are a form of ministry. Re-examine the motives and priorities which lie behind what you do with your time. Let there be no sense of onerous duty or guilt in this. There is no place for the tyranny of 'ought' in the scheme of love.

Action

Perform some small service, a little act of shepherding for someone you love, or for a plant or an animal. If you have a dog, give his bedding a good clean and if he is a shaggy creature, brush his coat.

Saturday in Easter Week

Reading

But the souls of the righteous are in the hand of God, and no torment will ever touch them. In the eyes of the foolish they seemed to have died, and their departure was thought to be a disaster, and their going from us to be their destruction; but they are at peace. For though in the sight of others they were punished, their hope is full of immortality. Having been disciplined a little, they will receive great good, because God tested them and found them worthy of himself; like gold in the furnace he tried them, and like a sacrificial burnt offering he accepted them. In the time of their visitation they will shine forth, and will run like sparks through the stubble. They will govern nations and rule over peoples, and the Lord will reign over them forever. Those who trust in him will understand truth, and the faithful will abide with him in love, because grace and mercy are upon his holy ones, and he watches over his elect (Wisd. 3:1–9 NRSV).

Meditation

This passage from the Wisdom of Solomon is usually read at a service for the commemoration of the dead, so it is easy to suppose that it is speaking only of the next life. But it is a pity to limit its meaning in this way, because the whole purpose of Christ's coming to us and of his dying and rising again is to make life in this world more vibrant and meaningful.

This in no way implies that we are to expect a trouble-free existence but that tribulation and torment will ultimately not harm those whose lives are hidden in Christ. Furthermore, without knowing how, they will shine forth, not by their own efforts or eloquence, but because of his light which shines forth from them. Truths are revealed to them, not as an intellectual 'eureka', but in the quietness of a heart which is capable of seeing with the uncluttered vision of childhood.

To those who want nothing to do with God, people who have elected him for themselves and been elected by him seem to have died. They are religious freaks, eccentrics not in touch with 'the real world'. But these eccentrics are at peace, not because they live in 'cloud cuckoo land', but because they look forward in the certainty which comes from experience to the consummation of the truth; the ultimate making good of all things.

This kind of election is a privilege available to everyone without exception. Dare to desire it for yourself.

Action

Do something to make 'life in this world more vibrant and meaningful' for yourself and those around you. A little thing will do, such as a change of routine, flowers on the table or a favourite meal.

First Sunday after Easter

Reading

So they drew near to the village to which they were going. He appeared to be going further, but they constrained him, saying, 'Stay with us, for it is toward evening and the day is now far spent.' So he went in to stay with them.

When he was at table with them, he took the bread and blessed, and broke it, and gave it to them. And their eyes were opened and they recognised him; and he vanished out of their sight. They said to each other, 'Did not our hearts burn within us while he talked to us on the road, while he opened to us the scriptures?' And they rose that same hour and returned to Jerusalem; and they found the eleven gathered together and those who were with them, who said, 'The Lord has risen indeed, and has appeared to Simon!' Then they told what had happened on the road, and how he was known to them in the breaking of the bread (Luke 24:28–35).

Meditation

So it is that God reveals himself silently and suddenly in our midst. Christ who is Lord of the impossible returns to his friends as one presumed dead. Place their feelings in the context of those whose sons return home from wars when they were presumed killed in action, or of brothers and sisters reunited after forty years of separation brought on by the Nazi holocaust. Earlier on, the disciples had expressed a rather wistful hope that Jesus was the one destined to redeem Israel but as he points out to them the necessity of all that he has been through, their hearts begin to burn within them.

If something is necessary it implies some sort of sequel to the event. The breaking of the bread leads to more than physical revelation. It is a moment of instant and irrevocable recognition of an eternal truth and of the full meaning of the Resurrection for the world. It is over almost instantly, as such moments always are, because they cannot be deliberately prolonged or expressed in words. They belong to the pure in heart and to young children, who often understand from the heart the meaning and purpose of existence.

Desire purity of heart with which to see and know the risen Christ in a rushed and crowded world and to glean new truths from the reading of scripture, as well as from literature and poetry that are not specifically sacred.

Action

Break some bread and share a glass of wine with one or two other people, conscious of Christ's presence among you. You could centre the action around this prayer. It is the Collect which is said on Saturday night at Compline:

As the watchman looks for the morning, even so do our eyes wait for you, O Christ. Come with the dawning of the day, and make yourself known to us in the breaking of the bread, for you are the Risen Lord, for ever and ever.

Saint Athanasius
2 May

Reading

Now the Catholic Faith is this: that we worship one God in
Trinity and the Trinity in Unity; Neither confusing the Persons:
nor dividing the Substance. For there is one person of the Father;
another of the Son and another of the Holy Spirit. But the
Godhead of the Father, of the Son, and of the Holy Spirit is one:
the glory equal, the Majesty co-eternal.

From the Athanasian Creed

Meditation

The *Concise Oxford Dictionary*'s definition of the word
'catholic' reads as follows: 'Universal; of interest or use to
all; all-embracing, of wide sympathies, broad-minded, toler-
ant'. While the Church through the ages has not always lived
up to its catholicity, God is all of these things and more.

We limit our experience of God and impoverish our faith by
fearfully clinging to outmoded language and to ways of
thinking of the Creator and of ourselves in relation to God,
which either exclude many people or make them feel inferior.
Fearful and rigid adherence to dogma is a great excluder and
the imagination is the free gift of God's Spirit, who is the great
inspirer and motivator of the artist and thinker in every
human being.

The idea of the Trinity is a source of great freedom and of
endless possibility. Far too much has been said about it and
very few people have come close to experiencing from the

heart that glory and co-eternal majesty which is beyond words; so here is a story which appeared in our parish magazine and which comes closer to defining the mystery of the Trinity than some of the most learned treatises on the subject.

A Sunday school teacher had spent about fifteen minutes trying to explain to the children what the doctrine of the Trinity was all about. After her explanations she sent them off into the churchyard with instructions to find and draw things in their surroundings that would symbolise the Trinity. She was duly presented with some of the more predictable images; the cross, the wind, sunshine, etc., when David, aged nine, showed her his drawing (reproduced below). He explained

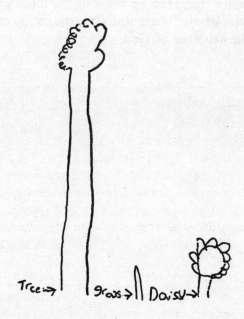

that the tree was very big and strong, like the Father. He then said that when he looked at the grass he realised that each blade was just like the others which reminded him of Jesus, the Son, who had come to be just like us. He then went on to explain that he had drawn a daisy because it filled him with joy like that of the Holy Spirit.

Jesus said: 'Whoever does not receive the Kingdom of God like a child will never enter it'. Give free rein to your imagination and desire fresh insight into the nature of the Godhead.

Action

Ask a young child to describe to you the idea of the Trinity or of anything relating to the Christian faith which you perhaps find obscure.

To balance this, read up some of the theology which has been developed over the centuries on the nature of the Trinity and on the existence of God.

Julian of Norwich
8 May

Reading

*He showed me a little thing, the size of a hazelnut, in the palm of
my hand, and it was as round as a ball. I looked at it with my
mind's eye and I thought, 'What can this be?' And answer came,
'It is all that is made.' I marvelled that it could last, for I thought
it might have crumbled to nothing, it was so small. And the
answer came into my mind, 'It lasts and ever shall because God
loves it.' And all things have being through the love of God.*

*In this little thing I saw three truths. The first is that God
made it. The second is that God loves it. The third is that God
looks after it.*

*What is he indeed that is maker and lover and keeper? I cannot
find words to tell. For until I am one with him I can never have
true rest nor peace. I can never know it until I am held so close to
him that there is nothing in between.*

From *The Revelations Of Divine Love*

Meditation

Dame Julian's 'showings' were given to her during the course
of a severe illness. They were not visions which she saw with
her eyes, but understandings of various aspects of the mystery
of God and of his love for the human race. She was a
fourteenth-century mystic, but the great gifts which were
given to her in prayer, and to others like her, are still being
proffered to us today.

In the modern world, we need more than ever to experience

God, rather than merely to read books about him or address long-winded and flowery prayers to him, to which we seldom listen for an answer.

Prayer is about listening, longing and waiting. One thing only is needful, the recognition of the need itself. Dame Julian received these truths as they were laid upon her heart, because she had first learned to wait open-heartedly for them to be given to her. Prayer which leads to the ultimate union of which she speaks is a gift of God's Spirit. It is not something which is earned or worked at. It is a gift which is often bestowed on the most unlikely people. There is not a single person in the world who is deserving of it.

Spend a few minutes being still and centred from the heart, all the time loving and desiring a closer union with God. The prayer for Tuesday in Passion Week on page 154 is a good way in to this exercise, but before praying it, take the time consciously to place yourself in God's presence, using any kind of aid which the imagination may supply you with, such as imagining yourself standing before God and his angels in heaven. Be conscious of his love for you and of the fact that his love does not change or go away, regardless of your actions or moods. Own and be thankful for the good aspects of your personality, as well as your talents and attributes and realise that they are given to you as free gifts by the God who loves you.

Action

Go for a walk and take home something large or small which will be a reminder of what happened during the prayer time.

Saint Gregory of Nazianzen
9 May

Reading

*While staying here I accompany you in love, for affection makes
everything common between us.*

Letter to Gregory of Nyssa

Meditation

Gregory of Nazianzen, a fourth-century Father of the Church
spent much of his life contending with the consequences of the
Arian heresy, a view which basically challenged the nature of
Christ in the Godhead. The heresy was refuted and Christ's
relationship to the Father defined as 'consubstantial' by the
Council of Nicea in AD 325, a few years before Gregory was
born.

In the early days of the Church much energy, and even life,
was expended on what was deemed to be heretical. In fourth
century Cappadocia, where Gregory was born, theology was
as normal a topic of conversation as politics or the state of the
economy are today. But even today the Christian Church is
still torn apart by questions of dogma, although there are
many people searching for a way forward together in a spirit
of Christian love. The difficulties presented by the importance
of defining what we actually believe, as opposed to making our
one priority the desire to live Christ's love in the world, seem
insurmountable.

Christ did not come to bring peace, but a sword. There is no
escaping conflict. The cross itself symbolises both a meeting

and a juxtaposition of two opposing forces. Christ, the Incarnate God of love, places himself at the heart of all conflict and makes our common love for him the means whereby we can hold all things intellectual and spiritual in common.

Action

Here is a recipe for elderflower champagne. It takes a week or ten days to mature:

INGREDIENTS

4 elderflower heads in full bloom
$4\frac{1}{2}$ litres (1 gallon) cold water
1 lemon
700g ($1\frac{1}{2}$lb) loaf sugar
2 tablespoons white vinegar

Dissolve the sugar in a little warm water and allow to cool. Squeeze the juice from the lemon, cut the rind in four, put the pieces with the elderflowers in a large jug or basin, add the wine vinegar and pour on the rest of the cold water. Leave to steep for 4 days. Strain off and bottle in screw-topped bottles. It should be ready to drink in 6 to 10 days but test after 6 days to see that it does not get too fizzy. If it fails to work, leave it for another week; sometimes the natural yeast of the flowers is very slow to get going and occasionally you will get a batch which fails altogether. Serve chilled or with ice and lemon.

Second Sunday after Easter

Reading

The thief comes only to steal and kill and destroy; I came that they may have life, and have it abundantly (John 10:10).

Meditation

A life which is in Christ and filled with the creative energy of his Holy Spirit amounts to more than a code of behaviour and diligently attending church on Sundays. God wants more than anything that we should be united to him in the fullness of the joy of living. We were created to be happy. All of life is a gift from God to be enjoyed and shared with him in gratitude. A good meal, making love, a laugh, a really absorbing book or film, all of these things are his gifts to us.

The thief comes to take joy out of our lives by distorting it. He creeps up on fun and turns it into duty. Joy becomes boredom, often laced with fear. There is nothing so sad as a bored teacher trying to instill in the minds of children information which he or she finds boring or irrelevant. Sad, too, are the relationships where individuals share a house but live life as if it was a penance. A good row, like a good thunderstorm can be a breath of fresh air in a marriage, as long as the point of dispute is fully resolved and real reconciliation takes place between all parties concerned.

The Lord, the giver of life, must be invited into every aspect of daily existence, that he who is Lord of the Dance may dance with us in it. Even in times of personal suffering his dance, the great gift of life, is going on all around us. Young leaves, young animals, new plants taking root for the summer – even weeds – all of these affirm the new covenant and the rich complexity of life which is ours. When our own personal lives are in darkness and turmoil new life is always being secretly created, as new and abundant life is brought forth from the darkness of the earth.

Action

Do something which you normally enjoy doing with abandon and with fullness of joy. Do it in a way which joins you and the action to God in a spirit of gratitude and great love.

Here is a recipe for cheese fondu which is eaten out of one pot into which everyone dips. It is a good meal to have as a celebration of the togetherness of family life. Ideally, it should be accompanied by schnapps, but if this is not available, open a bottle of good white wine instead.

Fondu is traditionally cooked in a copper pot, but this is not essential. However, the pot must be capable of withstanding the heat of a flame or electric ring. The cheese needs to keep on bubbling while it is being eaten or it will very quickly turn into chewing gum!

INGREDIENTS FOR 4

225g (8oz) of Gruyère cheese
225g (8oz) of Emmental cheese (allow 100–125g (4oz) of cheese per head)
1 tbsp of cornflour (enough for up to 6 people)
½ bottle of dry white wine
¼ glass of kirsch (depending on taste)
A large clove of garlic
Grated nutmeg
Freshly ground black pepper

Combine the Gruyère, Emmental and cornflour in a large bowl. Rub the fondu pot with a generous amount of garlic.

Place the pot over a medium flame or electric ring set on medium and put the cheese and cornflour mixture in it.

Slowly add white wine and stir until you have a smooth mixture.

Add the grated nutmeg, the freshly ground black pepper and the kirsch.

Allow the mixture to bubble gently (about 5 mins) while you slice a baguette of french bread into small pieces to be put on the end of skewers and dipped into the fondu. Serve immediately.

Cheese fondu is very good served with a green salad and followed by a light refreshing mixture of oranges and lychees, with a little fresh mint mixed in. Tinned lychees are easily obtained in most supermarkets.

Third Sunday after Easter

Reading

O Lord, thou art my God; I will exalt thee, I will praise thy name; for thou hast done wonderful things, plans formed of old, faithful and sure. On this mountain the Lord of hosts will make for all peoples a feast of fat things, a feast of wine on the lees, of fat things full of marrow, of wine on the lees well refined. And he will destroy on this mountain the covering that is cast over all peoples, the veil that is spread over all nations. He will swallow up death for ever, and the Lord God will wipe away tears from all faces, and the reproach of his people he will take away from all the earth; for the Lord has spoken. It will be said on that day, 'Lo, this is our God; we have waited for him, that he might save us. This is the Lord; we have waited for him; let us be glad and rejoice in his salvation' (Isa. 25:1, 6–9).

Meditation

Here is an illustration of the way in which we are mothered by God, for God is both mother and father to all. There is not a single moment or aspect of any living thing, down to the smallest atom or molecule which is not suffused in his love, for he continues to love the world into being. The covering and the veil are what prevent people from experiencing God as mother and as father. They stifle hope, that ability to look forward with certainty to the good things which lie ahead. Hope comes from being already conscious and grateful for the good things of today.

Darkness is not knowing God. But darkness also serves a purpose, like protective clothing or sunglasses, because at present his glory would be too great for us to bear. God is unknowable and the mystery of his motherhood and father-hood unfathomable, like very deep, still water which by virtue of its depth and stillness makes it safe to swim in. The swimmer is so small in comparison to the depth of the water, he or she is held up and protected by its deepness.

We wait from the deepest part of ourselves for God, our mother and our father. We were created to wait for God. Deep answers deep. He is hidden in our midst and at the heart of every individual on earth so 'Let us be glad and rejoice in his salvation'.

Action

Rupert Brooke in his poem, 'These I have loved', speaks of 'the benison (blessing) of hot water'. Have a hot bath and experience in its all-embracing warmth, the enfolding love of God.

Fourth Sunday after Easter

Reading

Jesus said, 'Set your troubled hearts at rest. Trust in God always; trust also in me. There are many dwelling-places in my Father's house; if it were not so I should have told you; for I am going there on purpose to prepare a place for you. And if I go and prepare a place for you, I shall come again and receive you to myself, so that where I am you may be also; and my way there is known to you.' Thomas said, 'Lord, we do not know where you are going, so how can we know the way?' Jesus replied, 'I am the way; I am the truth and I am life; no one comes to the Father except by me' (John 14:1–7 NEB).

Meditation

Resting and trusting amount to the same thing. When children learn to swim they begin to learn only from the moment they cease to thrash about in the water and rest quietly in the hands of their teacher. When we cease thrashing about in life and learn to rest in God and to rest all the things which touch us in God, the incoherent and perplexing problems which beset us begin to take on meaning and direction. Resting in God, especially in times of stress, prevents drowning.

Life and prayer are bound up in each other. They are correspondent and interdependent, a sort of balancing act like learning to ride a bicycle. The hand or the extra little wheels are there to steady and to guide, but once children have learned the art of balancing they no longer need these outward aids because they have become built in.

Christ is the balance as well as the guiding and controlling hand which, as a person grows in him, become inner strength and peace and the way forward to eternal life.

Action

Experience trust in some tangible way. You could go for a bicycle ride, or teach a child to ride one or to swim. Or else try learning to ice-skate if there is a rink near you, or for the really intrepid, gliding or hang-gliding. Anything in which the experience of the teacher's skill and support become your own strength illustrates how Christ has made himself the way, the truth and life itself for us.

Our Lady, Help of Christians
21 May

Reading

Hail, Mary, full of grace: the Lord is with thee: blessed art thou among women, and blessed is the fruit of thy womb (Luke 1:28, 42).

Meditation

Encounter Mary and the Christ-child. Ask her to allow you to hold him. Feel the weight of his body against yours and the quality of his hair and skin. Let a dialogue build up between you and him, or between you and his mother, but don't force anything. Wait for the Lord to be with you. Wait for the moment to happen naturally.

See Mary in whatever way she presents herself to you, not necessarily as an ethereal young girl, but perhaps, which is more likely, as a strong woman of the country with clear intelligent eyes. Notice her hands as they hold and caress the child. They are more likely to be the hands of a woman who knows the meaning of physical work, rather than the delicate hands of the maidens portrayed by artists through the centuries. Palestinian women are strongboned and handsome to this day.

Allow this woman, who has suffered the ultimate possible for a mother to suffer, to speak to you about yourself, about your relationship with a child or with your own mother or mother-in-law.

Action

If you know a single parent or one who is tied to a house and young children, offer to babysit for a few hours. See and experience the Christ-child in the children you look after.

Rogation Sunday
Fifth Sunday after Easter

Reading

The Lord is near to all who call on him, to all who call on him in truth (Ps. 145:18 NRSV).

Meditation

The Latin verb from which the word 'rogation' is derived means to ask for a need to be fulfilled. Christ is not only near in times of need but present in the need itself, especially in times of doubt and despair. There is no human experience that he has not already met, for he was fully human and fully God and his human life was as beset with doubts, fears and frustrations as anyone else's.

He allowed himself to be constrained by the circumstances and people of his own time and meets those same constraints with us today. There is no agony of mind that he has not experienced and because we are caught up in him and a part of him, there is nothing of us that he does not already know.

To call on the Lord in truth, therefore, is to reach out to him while fully owning one's doubt or fear or anger, knowing that it is already fully known and half way to being bought back.

The process of redemption, of being bought back from our own darkness begins with our asking, with our reaching out in the dark for the hand of God.

Action

Do you find it difficult to ask for help or receive a favour?
Once again make a point of letting someone know you need
them today (see p.88).

Ascension Day

Reading

'Men of Galilee, why do you stand looking into heaven? This Jesus, who was taken up from you into heaven, will come in the same way as you saw him go into heaven.' (Acts 1:11).

Meditation

In one of the side chapels of Wells Cathedral is a small bas-relief depicting the Ascension. It took me a couple of visits before I realised what it was meant to represent. My first impression was not so much of Christ being absorbed into mist and cloud or heavenly glory, as of a pair of feet disappearing through a couple of dozen hats which are being thrown into the air by the people standing below. The picture conveys all the excitement of a victorious football match or boat race. I could almost hear the cheers.

The Ascension is a season for cheering rather than looking backward with a sense of anticlimax. When the apostles had finished throwing their hats in the air, if they had them, they went down the mountain filled with joy and spent many hours praising God in the company of the other disciples and of Mary, the mother of Jesus.

Christ's Ascension is the triumphant affirmation of his Resurrection, the promise that he will come again in the way in which he departed. We have much hat-throwing and cheering to look forward to, so, if possible, let today be the occasion for the celebration of the triumph over death bequeathed to us by Christ, a triumph which cannot be taken from us, and of our anticipation of the place which is being prepared for us in our Father's house.

Action

Enjoy the elderflower champagne you made on the feast day of St Gregory of Nazianzen.

Sunday after Ascension Day

Reading

O that thou wouldst rend the heavens and come down, that the mountains might quake at thy presence – as when fire kindles brushwood and the fire causes water to boil – to make thy name known to thy adversaries, and that the nations might tremble at thy presence! When thou didst terrible things ... thou camest down, the mountains quaked at thy presence. From of old no one has heard or perceived by the ear, no eye has seen a God besides thee, who works for those who wait for him (Isa. 64:1–4).

Meditation

Anyone who has suffered injustice, knows what it feels like to wait for wrongs to be put right. The apparently trifling injustices of day to day existence are all too familiar to most of us – the unfair parking ticket, the preferential treatment of a colleague or classmate, days when everything seems to be going against us and when it would have been better to have stayed in bed. There are also long-term and deeply-felt injustices, received at the hands of friends, relatives or society itself.

All of these things get under the skin and build up anger; but Christ has made his name known to our adversaries. Our own anger and desire for revenge are irrelevant in the face of his power because his perception of the truth is so much greater than ours.

There are many people who allow their lives to be consumed

by anger. They live to rail against fate. Human anger fuels itself and destroys at the same time, but the apocalyptic coming of the Saviour and his daily coming in our lives consume only what is irrelevant and hurtful to his creation. His consuming fire reveals the true context of a situation and he restores all things to their rightful place so that understanding and compassion can be brought out of confusion and hatred.

When the lens of a camera is focused correctly, the picture suddenly becomes clear. Its truth is made plain. God's judgment consists in demonstrating the truth, and in revealing the heart of the individual and the heart of a nation or society. In a single moment we shall understand. We are not to speculate on the punishment of those who wrong us because we have no idea of the extent of their own private suffering. All suffering is utterly lonely. We do not know what is happening in the hearts of other people or in the heart of a nation, but God's mercy is infinite and beyond our understanding. In praying for those who do us wrong we begin from a place of strength, the strength of the Father, the Creator God, Christ our brother who sees and understands the truth in every injustice.

Action

If there is someone who has wronged you, or if there is a group of people of whom you have a particular fear or dislike, try getting into their skin, as it were. Leaving aside whatever it is that stands between you, try to experience what it feels like to be that person or a member of that group.

PENTECOST

Whitsunday

Reading

When the day of Pentecost had come, they were all together in one place. And suddenly a sound came from heaven like the rush of a mighty wind, and it filled all the house where they were sitting. And there appeared to them tongues as of fire, distributed and resting on each one of them. And they were all filled with the Holy Spirit and began to speak in other tongues, as the Spirit gave them utterance.

Now there were dwelling in Jerusalem Jews, devout men from every nation under heaven. And at this sound the multitude came together, and they were bewildered, because each one heard them speaking in his own language. And they were amazed and wondered, saying, 'Are not all these who are speaking Galileans? And how is it that we hear, each of us in his own native language? Parthians and Medes and Elamites and residents of Mesopotamia, Judea and Cappadocia, Pontius ... Egypt and the parts of Libya belonging to Cyrene, and visitors from Rome, both Jews and proselytes, Cretans and Arabians, we hear them telling in our own tongues the mighty works of God.' (Acts 2:1–11).

Meditation

Language both divides and unites. As a speaker of more than one language I can personally vouch for the joys of being able to communicate with people who are not of one's own cultural background. If you speak someone else's language you understand in some measure what makes that person 'tick'. The more fluently you speak their language, the more you are able to empathise with a people as a whole, as well as with a given individual. The gift of empathy and communication is the provenance of God's Holy Spirit who is the *pneuma*, the breath of life, the enabler.

The miracle of Pentecost was not only a miracle of speaking but of understanding. It was a miracle of communication and therefore of peace. We are brought, through Christ's Spirit, out of the chaos of Babel into this life-giving fire of understanding, for it is understanding which enables nations, communities, churches and families to be re-created, so that they in turn can re-create our world.

Action

Do something which challenges insularity or parochial attitudes. Try learning a new language or brushing up one you already know. Read a newspaper or book which does not represent your particular point of view. Read it in a spirit of seeking to understand what it is that makes people think differently from you and try to find some common ground, no matter how small, on which to build for the future.

The Feast of Weeks
Shavuoth

Reading

As I looked, behold, a stormy wind came out of the north, and a great cloud, with brightness round about it, and fire flashing forth continually, and in the midst of the fire, as it were gleaming bronze (Ezek. 1:4–8).

From the prophetic readings used in the Synagogue
on the first day of the Feast of Weeks

Meditation

The Jewish Feast of Weeks, or *Shavuoth*, falls on the fiftieth day after Passover and coincides roughly with our own Pentecost. It commemorates God's revelation of his law in the giving of the commandments on Mount Sinai. At Pentecost the disciples were fired with courage and love by God's Spirit who enabled them and their descendants to reveal the new covenant which had been sealed and ratified in the sacrifice of God's Son. The Jewish feast is also one of thanksgiving for the first harvest. Its Hebrew name, *Shavuoth*, signifies a bringing together and a celebration of fruitfulness.

In desiring to know God better we are moved by love to desire to keep his law, in other words to order our lives in keeping with the great commandment of love. The new covenant bequeathed to us in Christ has too often been understood as a bleak moral code, rather than the fruits of a simple desire to be more fully conformed to his image and

229

likeness in our thinking and feeling, as well as in our doing.

Let today be a day of thanksgiving for the good things of summer, for warmth or rain and for abundance of vegetation. Let the sunshine and summer skies be a reminder of God's covenant and the wind the all-encompassing presence of the Holy Spirit. Let it be a day of inner celebration and wonder.

Action

Dairy dishes such as cheese blintzes are normally eaten during *Shavuoth*. Here is a recipe:

INGREDIENTS

for the batter:
    1 cup of sifted all-purpose flour
    1 tsp salt
    4 eggs, well beaten
    1 cup of milk or water

INGREDIENTS

for the filling:
    700g (1½lb) of dry cottage cheese
    1 or 2 egg yolks, beaten
    1 tbsp of melted butter
    Salt, sugar and cinnamon to taste

Sift the flour and salt. Mix the eggs with the liquid and stir in the flour. Mix until smooth to form thin batter. Pour on to a hot, lightly-greased small skillet enough batter to form a very thin cake, tilting the pan from side to side so that the batter spreads evenly. Turn out on to a clean cloth, cooked side up. Allow to cool. Repeat until all the batter is used.

For the filling: mix the cheese with the egg yolks and butter and with salt, sugar and cinnamon to taste. Place a tablespoon of the mixture in the centre of each cake. Fold the edges over to form an envelope. Blintzes may be prepared and filled in advance and kept in the refrigerator until ready to fry. Just before serving, fry them in butter until brown on both sides, or bake in a moderate oven. Serve hot with sour cream, or with a sugar and cinnamon mixture. Makes about 10 blintzes.

Saint Columba
9 June

Reading

Thursday of Columba benign,
Day to send sheep on prosperity,
Day to send cow on calf,
Day to put the web in the warp.

Day to put coracle on the brine,
Day to place the staff to the flag,
Day to bear, day to die,
Day to hunt the heights.

Day to put horses in harness,
Day to send herds to pasture,
Day to make prayer efficacious,
Day of my beloved, the Thursday,
           Day of my beloved, the Thursday.
         Celtic prayer from the *Carmina Gadelica*

Meditation

Columba's feast day is traditionally kept on a Thursday and
this Celtic prayer, which is dedicated to him, illustrates how
the crofters of Scotland and Ireland centred their lives on God.
Every action and every moment of the day were consecrated to
God in words or songs of praise and supplication. Children
were raised strong in the belief that they and all human
beings were part of a great living organism whose separate

constituents were given over to the adoration of God, each with its place in the great eternal Order of creation, alongside Mary, the angels, human beings on earth and all the saints in heaven. They were taught that it was unnatural *not* to pray.

The songs and poetry of those early Christians reveal how the habit of prayer, instilled in the young from the moment that they were first rocked and nursed by their mothers, was as necessary to life as air or food.

Use this time to own more fully your personal need for God. Is prayer becoming a necessary habit, not just an onerous duty? Is God becoming a place of refuge and a source of inspiration and energy? Do you set aside a regular time and place each day to be alone with him? Are there times in the day when you quickly and almost unconsciously reach for him?

If you have time, take into your inner space the many millions of people whose lives are governed by the need to survive in a materialistic and competitive world and who do not know how to be inwardly still.

Action

Take a routine action, such as washing-up, and consecrate it in God. If the Holy Spirit inspires you, write a short prayer or poem which can be said every day as you do this particular job.

Saint Benno
16 June

Reading

Bless the Lord, seas and rivers,
sing praise to him and highly exalt him for ever.
Bless the Lord, you whales and all
creatures that move in the waters,
sing praise to him and highly exalt him for ever.
Bless the Lord, all birds of the air,
sing praise to him and highly exalt him for ever.
Bless the Lord, all beasts and cattle,
sing praise to him and highly exalt him for ever

Meditation

Saint Benno is one of the lesser known early Celtic saints. I
have included him for two reasons. First, out of affection for
all children with the name of Ben and second, because the
following story which is told of the Saint seems fitting for this
time of year when the noises of the countryside are often far
from peaceful.

Benno was a holy man, much given to solitary walks in the
fields, deep in prayer and meditation. On one occasion, when
he was walking by a certain bog, he was disturbed by the loud
croaking of a very talkative frog. He lectured it on the virtue of
silence, citing the frogs of Seraphus, who apparently never
croaked, as examples for him to follow. On hearing his stern
words the frog instantly fell silent. However, when Benno had

gone on a little farther he remembered the words of the three young men (quoted in today's reading) who praised God in the fiery furnace and he was overcome with remorse. He was also very much afraid that the croaking of the frogs might be more pleasing to God than his own thoughts and prayers, so he returned to the spot where he had been interrupted by the noisy frog and invited it to continue croaking and praising the Creator in its usual way. Whereupon the bog and surrounding fields were filled with the sound of all sorts of creatures giving praise to God by whatever means available to them.

Examine your attitudes to other people's style of worship, including those who belong to your own church.

Action

If you are a regular churchgoer, try visiting a different church this Sunday, perhaps one of another denomination. If you don't normally go to church, consider the idea of working through this book again with a group of other people. You could also make a few tentative investigations into a church or fellowship group which might suit you. The right church is worth travelling to. It doesn't have to be in your immediate neighbourhood.

Trinity Sunday
First after Pentecost

Reading

Now there was a man of the Pharisees, named Nicodemus, a ruler of the Jews. This man came to Jesus by night and said to him, 'Rabbi, we know that you are a teacher come from God; for no one can do these signs that you do, unless God is with him. Jesus answered him, 'Truly, truly, I say to you, unless one is born anew, he cannot see the kingdom of God.' Nicodemus said to him, 'How can a man be born when he is old? Can he enter a second time into his mother's womb and be born?' Jesus answered, 'Truly truly, I say to you, unless one is born of water and the Spirit, he cannot enter the kingdom of God. That which is born of the flesh is flesh, and that which is born of the Spirit is spirit. Do not marvel that I said to you, "You must be born anew"' (John 3:1–7).

Meditation

Newness and novelty are not the same thing. The word 'new', usually printed in large bright capitals and followed with a series of exclamation marks, is the clarion-call of the modern age. From the latest 'taste sensation' to today's trendy electronic gadget, which will be replaced next month with something still smaller and trendier, novelty in newness is what counts.

At least Nicodemus understood that the sort of newness of which Jesus was speaking had nothing to do with built-in obsolescence. But what he found inconceivable was the idea of complete transformation and new beginning, rather than the updating of something already in existence.

The new beginning which was under discussion is the gift of the Holy Spirit, the giver of life, who empowers the receiver to see the world through new eyes, to understand with a new and different intelligence and to love with a pure young heart. God's Spirit is unrepeatable newness, not the newness shouted in the shifting messages of commercial advertising, bewildering in its ultimate sameness. The newness of new life in Christ is whispered in the heart of a person who is made aware of the uniqueness of every human being – even of every living cell, for no two cells in the whole of creation are the same.

Baptism is the outward affirmation of our being made new in Christ and of the unrepeatable newness of creation.

Action

Light a candle this evening as a symbol of your baptism through which you have been brought out of darkness into light. You can also celebrate your membership in the Christian family with some sugared almonds, which are traditionally eaten at christenings. Here is a recipe:

EQUIPMENT

    1 large heavy saucepan
    1 metal tablespoon
    1 wooden spoon
    1 sieve

INGREDIENTS

    450g (1lb) granulated sugar
    100/125ml (4 fl oz) water
    1 tsp cinnamon
    450g (1lb) almonds with their skins on

Put the sugar and water into the saucepan and dissolve slowly over low heat, stirring all the time with the tablespoon. Add the cinnamon, stir, raise the heat and then boil until the syrup falls in thick drops from the spoon.

Remove from the heat, add the almonds and stir until they are well coated with the syrup. Continue stirring until the syrup dries to sugar. Remove the almonds.

Put the excess sugar back into the pan, add a little water and dissolve. Boil until the syrup clears, add the once-coated almonds and stir until they are coated a second time with the syrup. Cool. If you are not going to eat them straight away, pack them in jars with airtight stoppers or lids.

Second Sunday after Pentecost

Reading

'I am the true vine, and my Father is the vinegrower. He removes every branch in me that bears no fruit. Every branch that bears fruit he prunes to make it bear more fruit. You have already been cleansed by the word that I have spoken to you. Abide in me as I abide in you. Just as the branch cannot bear fruit by itself unless it abides in the vine, neither can you unless you abide in me. I am the vine, you are the branches. Those who abide in me and I in them bear much fruit, because apart from me you can do nothing' (John 15:1–5).

Meditation

Christ is all things to all people, as the stem of the vine is all things to the leaves and fruit which it sustains. Imagine that plants have a kind of free will in being disposed to grow or not. If a branch of the vine does not grow and bear fruit it may be that it is not disposed to do so. Its lack of willingness blocks off the life-giving sap which comes up from the main stem, so that it is no more than a stunted and barren parasite.

A living faith is not a crutch for the weak but the source of strength for those intrepid enough to risk living to the full. Christ is that source of strength which is still there for us to draw on, even in the context of modern living.

The word 'humility' has many different meanings, but it has its origins in the Latin *humus*, meaning soil. A plant must be rooted in the earth and disposed to receiving its nourishment from that source. We are rooted in Christ, or grafted on to him, so if we are to survive as human beings we need this kind of humility, which means not rejecting the nourishment he has to give us and even the pruning which must take place if we are to grow and bear fruit.

When the grapes have been harvested, the vine itself is cut down and left forlorn in the field, awaiting the growth of next year's grapes. Christ has allowed himself to be cut down and left forlorn, that we might reap the harvest of gladness of which we are an integral part.

Action

Open a bottle of wine tonight, or else enjoy some fresh grapes. A bunch of grapes is a very interconnected piece of vegetation, close-knit and compact, with each grape contributing to the graceful shape of the whole. The main stem of the bunch sustains the weight of all the little offshoots which are the grapes themselves.

You do not need to have a mature vine growing outside your door to appreciate our interdependence and oneness in Christ.

The Birth of Saint John the Baptist
24 June

Reading

*Now the time came for Elizabeth to be delivered, and she gave
birth to a son. And her neighbours and kinsfolk heard that the
Lord had shown great mercy to her, and they rejoiced with her.
And on the eighth day they came to circumcise the child; and
they would have named him Zechariah after his father, but his
mother said, 'Not so; he shall be called John.' And they said to
her, 'None of your kindred is called by this name.' And they
made signs to his father, inquiring what he would have him
called. And he asked for a writing tablet, and wrote, 'His name is
John.' And they all marvelled. And immediately his mouth was
opened and his tongue loosed, and he spoke, blessing God. And
fear came on all their neighbours. And all these things were
talked about through all the hill country of Judea; and all who
heard them laid them up in their hearts, saying, 'What then will
this child be?' For the hand of the Lord was with him. And the
child grew and became strong in spirit, and he was in the
wilderness till the day of his manifestation to Israel*

(Luke 1:57–66, 80).

Meditation

When I was at my convent preparatory school, one day a year
(it was always in the summer term and the sun always shone)
was reserved for what was called the Great Feast. We were
never told when it was going to be. It was simply announced at
morning assembly or disguised as a fire drill. Lessons were

cancelled and the day was instantly transformed into a holiday which was packed with games and treats and topped with strawberries and cream, the crowning glory of an enormous summer tea.

Right until the day itself, we relished the inevitability of the coming of the Great Feast, and yet it always came when it was least expected. Our headmistress would sometimes begin the day by saying in a stern and sombre tone of voice that she had something very serious to tell us, and then she would announce the Great Feast.

The birth and naming of John the Baptist and the feelings which these events evoked among his relatives and the close friends of the family correspond to what we felt when the bell rang on the morning of the Great Feast and while Mother Magdalen John was making her announcement – a mixture of excitement and trepidation.

It is exactly six months until Christmas, so we relish with quiet excitement the coming of God's gift of himself to the world.

Action

Now is about the right time to start making Christmas pudding, so here is a time-honoured family recipe, slightly embellished:

INGREDIENTS

225g (8oz) shredded suet
1 heaped tsp of mixed spice
$\frac{1}{2}$ tsp of grated nutmeg
$\frac{1}{4}$ tsp of ground cinnamon
100g/125g (4oz) plain flour
100g/125g (4oz) soft brown sugar
100g/125g (4oz) white breadcrumbs grated from a stale loaf
175g (6oz) sultanas

175g (6oz) raisins
175g (6oz) currants
50g (2oz) almonds blanched, skinned and chopped
50g (2oz) mixed peel finely chopped, whole candied and
    citron peel (if available)
The grated rind and juice of 1 lemon
14 tsp salt
4 standard eggs
150ml (5 fl oz) barley wine, stout, milk or orange juice
2 tsp rum

Mix the suet, sugar, flour and breadcrumbs. Clean the fruit and chop the raisins. Add all the fruit, including the almonds, as well as the spices, peel, lemon rind and salt. Mix these dry ingredients thoroughly together. Strain in the lemon juice and add the beaten eggs, rum and other juices.

Cover the bowl with a cloth and let it stand for a few hours or overnight. Grease 2 pudding basins and pack the mixture into them right to the top. Cover each basin with a square of greaseproof paper. Tie the paper on to the rims of the bowls with string. Steam the puddings for 8 hours. Store in a cool dry place until Christmas when they should be steamed for a further 2 hours.

Third Sunday after Pentecost

Reading

When one of those who sat at table with him heard this, he said to him, 'Blessed is he who shall eat bread in the kingdom of God!' But he said to him, 'A man once gave a great banquet, and invited many; and at the time for the banquet he sent his servant to say to those who had been invited, "Come; for all is now ready." But they all alike began to make excuses. The first said to him, "I have bought a field, and I must go out and see it; I pray you, have me excused." ... And another said, "I have married a wife, and therefore I cannot come." So the servant came and reported this to his master. Then the householder in anger said to his servant, "Go out quickly to the streets and lanes of the city, and bring in the poor and maimed and blind and lame." And the servant said, "Sir, what you commanded has been done, and still there is room." And the master said to the servant, "Go out to the highways and hedges, and compel people to come in, that my house may be filled. For I tell you, none of those men who were invited shall taste my banquet"' (Luke 14:15–24).

Meditation

The conversation which immediately preceded this one concerned the sort of people to whom one ought to offer hospitality and the purpose of hospitality itself, which does not consist in being asked back or in being under any kind of obligation to give another even more expensive party in return. 'If that is the case' says the man sitting at table with

Jesus, 'the one who gets asked to your supper party is going to be lucky indeed' – presumably because, apart from anything else, that person will not have been required to present any social or economic credentials.

One of the Marx Brothers was once heard to say that he would never want to belong to a club which wanted someone like him as a member. Christ's banquet definitely lacks cachet. The most unsuitable people are invited to it, and the host is servant to the least attractive guest in a silent dialogue of mutual love. Any moment which is given over to the desire to meet God in this way is in reality a banquet of an extravagance beyond that of our wildest dreams.

Give a little more time to being alone with God today, in a spirit of desiring to respond to his invitation to the banquet.

Action

Invite some friends for a meal and include at least one person who has few friends or who you would not normally ask. Here is a recipe for Baked Aubergines (*Melanzane à la mozzarella*), as learned from my grandmother's Italian cook. It is an excellent supper dish, suitable for vegetarians.

INGREDIENTS

For 6 generous helpings

4 large aubergines
3 heaped tbsp of flour mixed with a little salt
Sunflower oil (you can, of course, use olive oil which gives the dish a more distinctive flavour but eggplants absorb a great deal, so I find it more economical to use sunflower oil)
225g (½lb) mozzarella cheese
2 tins of tomatoes (it helps to buy the ready chopped variety, or you can chop them yourself)

Italian herb seasoning or dried basil
sea salt and pepper

At least an hour before you want to begin cooking, slice the aubergines into 1cm ($\frac{1}{2}$in) slices. Sprinkle them lightly with salt and pile them in layers in a colander or sieve. Place a weighted plate on top of the pile of sliced aubergines and stand the colander where it can drain.

Pat the slices of aubergine dry with a paper towel and sprinkle them lightly with the flour and salt. Fry the slices for 2 or 3 minutes on each side in enough oil to cover the base of a large frying pan. You may need to top up the oil as you go along. Remove the slices from the oil when they are soft and lightly browned. Place them between layers of paper towels while you are waiting for the remaining ones to cook.

In a large oven dish, arrange alternate layers of cooked aubergine, 3 or 4 spoonfuls of tinned tomatoes, slices of mozzarella dotted over the surface, a small sprinkling of herbs and a little pepper. Be restrained with the salt.

When all the aubergines have been used, finish with a layer of tomato and a more generous amount of mozzarella. Bake in a moderate oven (180°C, 350°F Gas mark 4) for 20 minutes or until bubbling and brown on top.

Serve with rice, a green salad and a bottle of red wine.

Fourth Sunday after Pentecost

Reading

'Now before faith came, we were imprisoned and guarded under the law until faith would be revealed. Therefore the law was our disciplinarian until Christ came, so that we might be justified by faith. But now that faith has come, we are no longer subject to a disciplinarian, for in Christ Jesus you are all children of God through faith. As many of you as were baptized into Christ have clothed yourselves with Christ. There is no longer Jew or Greek, there is no longer slave or free, there is no longer male and female; for all of you are one in Christ Jesus. And if you belong to Christ, then you are Abraham's offspring, heirs according to the promise' (Gal. 3:23–end NRSV).

Meditation

Faith does not consist of blind belief in a set of disconnected and incomprehensible dictates issued by theologians and thinkers of the past. It is a gift from God, bestowed directly on the heart with the gentleness of summer rain. What we believe is what we know from having encountered and experienced God for ourselves now, in our own times. This is what is meant by 'living faith'. Spirituality is still couched in a great deal of jargon which can make it feel very exclusive, but experience of the risen Christ liberates us from every kind of isolation and from guilt and the onerous sense of duty which is associated with 'religion'. God is love, so faith which is not conceived and rooted in love is not faith. It is merely belief.

The law, or the commandments which were given to God's people in their infancy, served the same purpose as school rules. They enabled society to function and they schooled the individual in love and self-discipline. The coming of Christ in history affirms the maturity of his people. The coming of Christ in the life of the individual affirms that person's spiritual adulthood.

Freedom from set rules is not an invitation to anarchy but rather an invitation to harmonise with the Creator God in the music of life, both spiritual and temporal. Freedom from the law means freedom to allow the presence of the living God, rather than 'religion', to permeate every moment of living. No longer is God confined to Sundays and church. In fact he is quite often absent from both. He is with all human beings and for all human beings in every moment of daily life, so no one should cling to God or claim sole rights over him. He belongs to all. It is therefore up to every individual to respond to his invitation and at the same time to seek him out, each in their own way, as they are being continually sought out in the highways and hedges of last Sunday's parable.

Action

Next time it rains, go out and fully experience it. Don't wear waterproof clothing, just allow the rain to soak you. Warm summer rain, even if it is a downpour, is a good practical illustration of the soul encountering and experiencing the love of the living God.

If you have any plants growing indoors, check that they have plenty to drink. If it is a dry spell and you have a garden, tend the young plants, desiring their growth and well-being as you do so.

Saint Peter and Saint Paul
29 June

Reading

Now when Jesus came into the district of Caesarea Philippi, he asked his disciples, 'Who do people say that the Son of Man is?' And they said, 'Some say John the Baptist, but others Elijah, and still others Jeremiah or one of the prophets.' He said to them, 'But who do you say that I am?' Simon Peter answered, 'You are the Messiah, the Son of the living God.' And Jesus answered him, 'Blessed are you, Simon son of Jonah! For flesh and blood has not revealed this to you, but my Father in heaven. And I tell you, you are Peter, and on this rock I will build my church, and the gates of Hades will not prevail against it. I will give you the keys of the kingdom of heaven, and whatever you bind on earth will be bound in heaven, and whatever you loose on earth will be loosed in heaven.' Then he sternly ordered the disciples not to tell anyone that he was the Messiah (Matt. 16:13–20 NRSV).

Meditation

Here is another instance of living faith – God revealing himself in the heart of a person. Peter does not know that Christ is the Messiah because of what he has seen or been told. He knows with the instinctive knowledge which comes of having experienced the truth in love. This is what prompts him to speak.

All ministry is a matter of loving service. To minister means to tend or take care of someone. The keys of the kingdom are given to God's Church on earth to enable every single committed Christian to open doors through which others may pass in order to come closer to God. It is within the power of one who ministers to bestow immeasurable good, as well as immeasurable hurt. Whatever that person says or does in Christ's name stands. Whatever he or she refutes or puts down, whatever he or she inadvertently tramples on, cannot of itself be raised up. Ministry is an awesome responsibility.

When Jesus said that we, as God's Church, are built on a rock, he was not just playing with words. Even though we minister clumsily and cause hurt and misunderstanding; if we are prepared to return to the strength from which we came, the heart's knowledge of Christ, he who is our rock will enable reconciliation to take place and good to be brought forth from evil.

In this context, look at how you handle authority, particularly where it concerns helping others on their own spiritual journey.

Action

Give space in your heart where you encounter God for all those who are responsible for the spiritual well-being of others, especially for the ordained ministry.

There is much loneliness and unnoticed suffering among clergy. If you know of such a person, offer them real friendship. Imagine what you would like to have happen to you if you were in their predicament.

Fifth Sunday after Pentecost

Reading

Then someone came to him and said, 'Teacher, what good deed must I do to have eternal life?' And he said to him, 'Why do you ask me about what is good? There is only one who is good. If you wish to enter into life, keep the commandments.' He said to him, 'Which ones?' And Jesus said, 'You shall not murder; You shall not commit adultery; You shall not steal; You shall not bear false witness; Honour your father and mother; also, You shall love your neighbour as yourself.' The young man said to him, 'I have kept all these, what do I still lack?' Jesus said to him, 'If you wish to be perfect, go, sell your possessions, and give the money to the poor, and you will have treasure in heaven; then come, follow me.' When the young man heard this word, he went away grieving, for he had many possessions.

Then Jesus said to his disciples, 'Truly I tell you, it will be hard for a rich person to enter the kingdom of heaven. Again I tell you, it is easier for a camel to go through the eye of a needle than for someone who is rich to enter the kingdom of God.' When the disciples heard this, they were greatly astounded and said, 'Then who can be saved?' but Jesus looked at them and said, 'For mortals it is impossible, but for God all things are possible' (Matt. 19:16–26).

Meditation

Freedom from the law of rules and standards lies in total surrender. Surrender begins with a letting-go of the protective clothing which surrounds the person one is. The paradox of the Christian life lies in the fact that the less emotional protecting clothing one wears, the less vulnerable one is likely to be and in having less to protect we need less in the way of material possessions.

Possessions are not limited to material things or crude wealth. A possession might be a secure job which is unsuited to a person's real talent and therefore likely to prevent that person from following Christ with the heart and mind fully engaged. It might call for the letting go of a relationship which destroys or prevents growth. Surrender of possessions means letting go in the most complete way.

Christ is the light of the world. Our following of him has to be as single-minded as that of the young seedling which pushes up through the earth towards the source of life.

Letting go of possessions, both physical and personal, is a simultaneously active and passive process. We must live our lives open-handedly, or at least only lightly grasping the good things given to us, because all gifts, whether material or personal, are on loan from the Giver of life. We shall be held accountable for them, or perhaps we shall be required to return them today, so that even better things can be given to us tomorrow.

Action

Examine your attitude to your own possessions and to the way in which governments make use of wealth and resources. If you feel a need for change, act on it!

Mother Teresa of Calcutta

Reading

It is not how much we do that is pleasing to God, but how much love we put into the doing. Together let us build a chain of love around the world

Mother Teresa

Meditation

Mother Teresa's helpers are known by their simple blue-and-white habit, but not many people are aware of the invisible army of sick and suffering people who personally help the helpers and who further their work. Their help consists in allowing and accepting their own suffering with great love and even gratitude, so that the will of God can happen through them into the work of the Missionary Sisters of Charity.

Allowing love into one's life involves letting the most difficult moment or the simplest action be receptive to something greater than the immediate end in view. A meal which is prepared in love is a better-tasting meal than one which is thrown together in haste and indifference. For one thing, there are both the means and the time to allow all of the ingredients to give of their best.

There is no taste so good as fresh vegetables which have been lightly cooked, so as not to impair their flavour, and presented with love for those who will consume them, and with consideration for their natural beauty. Japanese food not only tastes delicious but looks delicious, because it is handled with love and consideration from the start.

What a person does in this spirit of cherishing and respecting of another person's value, or the intrinsic beauty of any living thing, no matter how small or insignificant the gesture, is a transferral of divine recreative energy. Be determined, therefore, to practise what in Buddhism is called 'mindfulness', the loving and full attention of the whole person to the present moment and the present task.

Action

Here is a recipe for a simple Japanese salad which, if prepared and presented with love, makes an excellent alternative to lettuce or tomato.

INGREDIENTS

275g (10oz) of Japanese radish (available in oriental grocery shops)
150g (5oz) carrots
1 tsp salt
½ cup vinegar
2 tbsp sugar
1 tbsp light soy sauce
½ tsp monosodium glutamate

Peel the radish, scrape the carrots and cut both into julienne strips. Salt lightly and allow to stand for thirty minutes. Press out the excess water with the hands, or pat dry with a clean cloth. Mix together the vinegar, sugar, soy sauce and monosodium glutamate. Carefully arrange the radish and carrot strips in a salad bowl, pour the dressing over them, mix lightly and serve.

Sixth Sunday after Pentecost

Reading

'Be merciful, just as your Father is merciful. Do not judge and you will not be judged; do not condemn and you will not be condemned. Forgive, and you will be forgiven; give, and it will be given to you. A good measure, pressed down, shaken together, running over, will be put into your lap; for the measure you give will be the measure you get back.'

He also told them a parable: 'Can a blind person guide a blind person? Will not both fall into a pit? A disciple is not above the teacher, but everyone who is fully qualified will be like the teacher. Why do you see the speck in your neighbour's eye, but do not notice the log in your own eye? Or how can you say to your neighbour, "Friend, let me take out the speck in your eye," when you yourself do not see the log in your own eye? You hypocrite, first take the log out of your own eye, and then you will see clearly to take the speck out of your neighbour's eye' (Luke 6:36–42 NRSV).

Meditation

Having taken the log out of our own eye, the chances are that we will no longer be interested in what is in our neighbour's. Our neighbour's fault will be quite irrelevant in comparison to his or her suffering. If I recognise my own inadequacy I cannot fail but recognise the absurdity of commenting on the same inadequacy in another person, because the things which irritate or outrage me the most in other people are often

255

those with which I have failed – knowingly or unknowingly – to come to terms with in myself.

God's mercy lies in his generosity. Mercy is another word for love, for we have not only been acquitted of our shortcomings, 'for there is no condemnation for those who are in Christ', but we have also been surrounded with a love which is so gentle and so constant that we seldom even notice it. It falls 'as the gentle dew from heaven'. Constant love has the same effect as soft rain. It gradually drenches other people's irritating habits. It can even override the sins of society because compassion is of divine, rather than human nature. God's love for us is unconditional and impartial. It is also given to us in such a way that we are empowered to pass it on intact to others and to all situations. We are all agents in the world's healing.

Action

Have a look at the things in other people or in a particular person which you feel most threatened by. Look at the things which threaten society as a whole – crime, Aids, the greed and selfishness which are destroying our environment – and allow from your own heart for God's mercy to fall on those situations and heal them.

The Feast of the Visitation
2 July

Reading

My soul magnifies the Lord, and my spirit rejoices in God my Saviour, for he has regarded the low estate of his handmaiden. For behold, henceforth all generations will call me blessed; for he who is mighty has done great things for me, and holy is his name. And his mercy is on those who fear him from generation to generation. He has shown strength with his arm, he has scattered the proud in the imagination of their hearts, he has put down the mighty from their thrones, and exalted those of low degree; he has filled the hungry with good things, and the rich he has sent empty away. He has helped his servant Israel, in remembrance of his mercy, as he spoke to our fathers, to Abraham and to his posterity for ever (Luke 1:46–55).

Meditation

My soul sings with adoration of you Lord, and I am filled with the gladness which comes from a sure knowledge of your presence. You have not despised me in my unworthiness. Instead, you have raised me up, so that others count me as highly favoured. For you, who are all powerful, have deigned to look with compassion upon me, the least of your servants. Blessed be your name forever, Lord. You love those who reverence your holy name, from generation to generation, throughout all time. When I am in need or in danger You are there to protect me. You have sent away those who imagine themselves to be important and you have brought down the rich and the powerful. Those who are of little account in the eyes of the world you have made to sit beside you and you have heaped honour on the poorest of your subjects. You have fed the hungry with good food – the living bread and wine of your love – and those who fancy they have no need of you, you have sent away empty handed and with empty hearts. You have kept your promise of mercy to the world, as you continue to speak through your prophets to this very day.

Make Mary's Magnificat your own by writing it out in terms that speak of yourself and of your own past.

Action

The Orthodox call Mary 'The Most Holy Theotokos' which means God-bearer. Pay someone a visit today, in a spirit of bringing Christ to them rather than with a view to 'converting' them.

Saint Mary Magdalene
22 July

Reading

But Mary stood weeping outside the tomb, and as she wept she stooped to look into the tomb; and she saw two angels in white, sitting where the body of Jesus had lain, one at the head and one at the feet. They said to her, 'Woman, why are you weeping?' She said to them, 'Because they have taken away my Lord, and I do not know where they have laid him.' Saying this, she turned round and saw Jesus standing, but she did not know that it was Jesus. Jesus said to her, 'Woman, why are you weeping? Whom do you seek?' Supposing him to be the gardener, she said to him, 'Sir, if you have carried him away, tell me where you have laid him, and I will take him away.' Jesus said to her, 'Mary.' She turned and said to him in Hebrew, 'Rabboni!' (which means Teacher). Jesus said to her, 'Do not hold me, for I have not yet ascended to the Father; but go to my brethren and say to them, I am ascending to my Father and your Father, to my God and your God.' (John 20:11–18).

Meditation

From death to life, from the darkness of the tomb to the light of day, from despair to hope realised and crowned with unutterable joy, from the remote and distant God of the mountain and of the Law to the intimate and personal God of love in Christ Jesus; all things are contained and all things are possible in the Lord of surprise.

'*Rabboni*' is an informal way of addressing a loved teacher.

In Arab countries a man of a certain age or station in life is addressed as '*Sidi*', which is also a term of endearment and is often used as a compliment. We too must greet the risen Christ, who is made manifest in every moment. We greet him like Mary, with unaffected love and confidence, recognising him as '*rabboni*', as '*sidi*', as friend and brother and desiring him for ourselves, in order that the world and every human being alive might have him more fully and know the Father as their own.

Christ brings us to the Father. By him and through him the Father is ours. By him and through him we are made his children with a place in his house which we can call our own, as our own children assume without questioning their right to a place at the family table.

Out of the man, Jesus, are revealed the power and glory of the omnipotent God. Revelation takes place at every level of existence, down to the minutiae of this present day, for there is infinite possibility for life and celebration in every moment which is taken up into Christ's Resurrection. His rising, our recognition of him and the gift of our new resurrected selves are like a party popper – so much colour, life and intricacy packed into such a tiny container – such celebration and surprise when the popper is popped.

Action

Recognise and greet Christ in someone when they come home today. Pop a few party poppers to celebrate the Resurrection.

Seventh Sunday after Pentecost

Reading

Therefore I have uttered what I did not understand, things too wonderful for me, which I did not know. I had heard of thee by the hearing of the ear, but now my eye sees thee; therefore I despise myself, and repent in dust and ashes (Job 42:3, 5, 6).

Depart from me, for I am a sinful man, O Lord (Luke 5:8).

Meditation

Both of these statements deal with the concept of human beings in relationship to God. They pertain to that moment in which we see ourselves in the context of his perfection and love. Such moments are times of great revelation, rather than inducements to feel guilty and grovel. They reveal how human beings have been touched and transformed from dust into something far more precious than the most valuable jewel in the world, while at the same time remaining a small earthy creature, infinitely loved and tenderly nurtured by the Creator.

The more we develop a relationship with God, without restricting the imagery we have of him, the more we realise our own littleness and the greatness of his and of her love. Relationship leads to dependence and need because this relationship, or dialogue which is called prayer, is one of a need being fulfilled and at the same time being made greater, so that the generosity of an all-powerful, loving God can be fully consummated in us. Prayer which is of the heart is a way of seeing and understanding, each according to our separate means, the nature of God. We arrive at a knowledge and loving acceptance of who God is and of who we are in that context. It is a dialogue which transcends words and images.

Hitherto Job had had a formal, almost theoretical, understanding of the maker of the universe, but he suddenly experiences a momentary glimpse of the Truth, a new dimension. Peter undergoes a similar kind of enlightenment, for it was not the miraculous catch of fish which he saw with his eyes which convinced him of the Divinity of Christ, but a word said softly in his heart which revealed to him the fullness of God's love.

Action

A few years ago the pop group 'UB 40' brought out a tape called 'I Got You Babe'. The song was originally sung in the sixties by Sonny and Cher. If you like pop music and can get hold of either the original record or the UB40 song, use them as a new way of deepening your relationship with the Lord. You could also listen to a favourite piece of classical music.

Eighth Sunday after Pentecost

Reading

For I tell you, unless your righteousness exceeds that of the scribes and Pharisees, you will never enter the kingdom of heaven.

You have heard that it was said to those of ancient times, 'You shall not murder'; and 'whoever murders shall be liable to judgment.' But I say to you that if you are angry with a brother or sister, you will be liable to judgment; and if you insult a brother or sister, you will be liable to the council; and if you say, 'You fool,' you will be liable to the hell of fire. So when you are offering your gift at the altar, if you remember that your brother or sister has something against you, leave your gift there before the altar and go; first be reconciled to your brother or sister, and then come and offer your gift (Matt. 5:20–4 NRSV).

Meditation

Letting go of pain is the beginning of forgiveness. Pain, however inflicted, is something which must be left at the altar of Calvary, while we allow the person or set of circumstances which have inflicted it to be brought into the embrace of God's healing and forgiveness.

This century has seen a great deal of pain. Recently there have been glimmers of hope for peace in the world where nations have been able to let go of past hurt, and to begin to free themselves from enslavement of one sort or another. In the former Eastern bloc countries, in South Africa, in relations between East and West and between rich and poor, knots of angry confrontation, injustice, inequality and the legacy of pain inherited from previous generations are slowly and gently being loosed.

Reconciliation is life itself. It is energy sparked off between two or three individuals to become the means for peace on a global scale. Anybody can be a part of this global reconciliation by desiring it from the heart and by spending a few minutes of each day acknowledging our own humanity and focusing our desire for peace into our experience of God.

Action

Be a peace-maker. Give some time to any group or organisation involved in the process of reconciliation or bridge-building between nations or groups of people. Do something to bring peace into a situation of conflict known to you, in your town, village or neighbourhood. There is still much to be done in the area of interdenominational dialogue. Be an ambassador for Christ and an agent of peace wherever you find yourself.

Ninth Sunday after Pentecost

Reading

Holy Father, keep them in thy name, which thou hast given me, that they may be one, even as we are one. While I was with them, I kept them in thy name, which thou hast given me; I have guarded them, and none of them is lost but the son of perdition, that the scripture might be fulfilled. But now I am coming to thee; and these things I speak in the world, that they may have my joy fulfilled in themselves. I have given them thy word; and the world has hated them because they are not of the world, even as I am not of the world. I do not pray that thou shouldst take them out of the world, but that thou shouldst keep them from the evil one. They are not of the world, even as I am not of the world. Sanctify them in the truth; thy word is truth. As thou didst send me into the world, so I have sent them into the world. And for their sake I consecrate myself, that they also may be consecrated in truth (John 17:11b–19).

Meditation

'We believe in one holy, catholic and apostolic Church' says the Creed. The words 'apostolic' and 'apostle' come from the Greek, *apostello*, meaning to send. An apostle is one who is sent out. We as the Church, the body of Christ and his apostles of today, are sent out into the world.

There is a big difference between being of the world and being in it. Those who are of the world are immersed in concerns which arise from principles and criteria incompatible with heaven, for heaven is, above all, the gratification of a consuming desire for God. People who are indifferent to God and who have no desire for that degree of 'sanctification' which will make them compatible with him will probably not feel comfortable in heaven. We go to the place to which we are best suited.

Being in the world, but not of it means seeking the reality of Heaven, what makes for real happiness, here and now 'in the land of the living' as the psalmist says, and conveying it in love to all people (see Ps. 27:13). Being in the world as apostles means desiring God and desiring perfection and purity of heart above all things, even at the cost of financial security or reputation.

Action

When you come to do your review of the day, have a look at your own priorities, without allowing the slightest tinge of guilt to creep in. You might find it helpful to finish with the prayer of abandonment.

The Transfiguration
6 August

Reading

For we did not follow cleverly devised myths when we made known to you the power and coming of our Lord Jesus Christ, but we had been eye-witnesses of his majesty. For he received honour and glory from God the Father when that voice was conveyed to him but the Majestic Glory, saying, 'This is my Son, my Beloved, with whom I am well pleased.' We ourselves heard this voice from heaven, while we were with him on the holy mountain. So we have the prophetic message more fully confirmed. You will do well to be attentive to this as to a lamp shining in a dark place, until the day dawns and the morning star rises in your hearts (2 Pet. 2:16–19 NRSV).

Meditation

Neither do we follow 'cleverly devised myths', although few of us have witnessed face to face the transparent glory of the living God. What some of us probably have witnessed, however, is the kind of glory which shines out of people who are wholly given over to God.

I know of an elderly nun (she is well over ninety) whom one would think had discovered the secret of eternal youth. She has the face of a young girl, with clear blue eyes which are full of wisdom and laughter. Whenever I am with her, I feel as though I am experiencing a revelation. She is a most gentle person and yet her face makes me think of apocalyptic descriptions of heaven – of crystal seas, angels with faces like the sun, and of jewels precious beyond price.

The Spirit of God can be contained in human beings to be revealed in moments of inexplicable happiness. Such is God's love and desire for us. Such is his humility. If we have the eyes with which to see and the ears to hear transfigured moments in time, as well as people transfigured by their love for God, the message of the gospel begins to make sense.

Religion is not an opiate or a myth, but a living reality which transfigures people and transforms lives.

Action

Be open to the possibility of being surprised by sudden joy or by a moment of profound understanding which cannot be expressed in words. Look at people, especially those close to you, in a spirit of readiness for God's radiance to be revealed to you in them.

Affirm this idea in something thoroughly practical, like cleaning a mirror or some windows, remembering that now 'we see through a glass darkly', or only catch occasional glimpses of the glory that is to come.

Tenth Sunday after Pentecost

Reading

'If then there is any encouragement in Christ, any consolation from love, any sharing in the Spirit, any compassion and sympathy, make my joy complete: be of the same mind, having the same love, being in full accord and of one mind. Do nothing from selfish ambition or conceit, but in humility regard others as better than yourselves. Let each of you look not to your own interests, but to the interests of others. Let the same mind be in you that was in Christ Jesus, who, though he was in the form of God, did not regard equality with God as something to be exploited but emptied himself, taking the form of a slave, being born in human likeness. And being found in human form, he humbled himself and became obedient to the point of death – even death on a cross. Therefore God also highly exalted him and gave him the name that is above every name, so that at the name of Jesus every knee should bend, in heaven and on earth and under the earth, and every tongue should confess that Jesus Christ is Lord, to the glory of God the Father' (Phil.2:1–11).

Meditation

The essence of humility lies in not getting in the way of love. It means not distracting someone from God with one's own 'persona' or with one's own selfish preoccupations. The most humble person is always the one whose heart, mind and will are most engaged in the service of others. Humility has nothing to do with grovelling and self-effacement. It has everything to do with a loving gratitude for the person I am and with a desire for others to rejoice in the people they are, that together we may reflect the multi-faceted glory of the living God.

All service is essentially creative and so complements the work of the Creator God who brings forth all things in love. A person who is engaged in any kind of creative work is an especially privileged servant, for pictures, poems and performances are all doorways. They are means whereby others can arrive at the truth. If the artist, writer or performer gets in the way of the work by imposing on it his or her own personality, he or she blocks the doorway through which those who are being served by the artist's work are eagerly waiting to pass.

Art and service are one and the same. The artist who is a servant and the servant who is an artist must listen to what the work wants to be. We obey the work. We do not subjugate it to ourselves.

Christ is both art and artist and the servant of servants. He is the way and the means whereby we pass through the door into a personal and immediate experience of the truth. We too are his works of art and the means whereby he rejoices in his creation. If we are not 'in full accord' and 'of one mind', we obstruct the work of creation and spoil the beauty of his workmanship. Being of one mind does not mean agreeing for the sake of peace and quiet, but seeking with all the gifts we hold in common to further the work of God's creation.

Action

Think about taking up some form of creative work and pursuing it in depth. There are any number of adult education courses in the visual arts, ranging from painting and ceramics to woodwork and embroidery. If you are mechanically minded, why not learn to service your own car? An engine, especially one that is in good working order, reflects the multifarious beauty of creation.

Saint Maximilian Kolbe
14 August

Reading

No one has greater love than this, to lay down one's life for one's friends (John 15:13 NRSV).

Meditation

Maximilian Kolbe was a Franciscan priest who gave his life for a fellow prisoner in the concentration camp of Auschwitz. The definition of martyr is 'witness', one whose life is given over as a statement of love for Christ and as an affirmation of Christ's love for the world. Maximilian gave his life in exchange for a man who was chosen to be starved to death, along with nine others, as a punishment for the escape of another inmate. The man in question had a wife and children and had pleaded with the guard for mercy.

When the SS men came to inspect the cell where the prisoners were left to die, they could not meet the clear penetrating gaze of the Franciscan whose face was transfigured by his love for Christ and for his fellow human beings.

Physical martyrdom is for the few, but the daily laying down of one's life for other people is within the reach of all. Members of a loving family experience martyrdom many times in a single day in countless moments of self-denial. A brother and sister who take turns and share toys without squabbling (even if only for half an hour!) are innocent witnesses to the love of Christ. Parents who willingly give of their time to support their child's school, or who endure hours of football in the pouring rain on a Saturday afternoon, are Christ-like in their loyalty and devotion. The parents of a handicapped child will experience martyrdom for the duration of that child's life, as will the man or woman given over to the care of an elderly person.

Witnessing with one's life means being given over entirely to the survival, well-being and happiness of another person. Anyone who is given over in love witnesses to the love of Christ and shares in his Passion, Resurrection and in his glory that is to come.

Action

If you know of someone who is experiencing martyrdom in daily life, do something practical to help them. There are people whose lives are entirely given over to the care of an elderly person or of a severely handicapped child or adult and who would be glad even of your company. If you know of someone like this, befriend them in some way. If not, seek them out through your church or local community service.

The Feast
of the Blessed Virgin Mary
15 August

Reading

*But when the fullness of time had come, God sent his Son, born
of a woman, born under the law, in order to redeem those who
were under the law, so that we might receive adoption as
children. And because you are children, God has sent the Spirit
of his Son into our hearts, crying 'Abba! Father!' So you are no
longer a slave but a child, and if a child then also an heir, through
God* (Gal. 4:4–7 NRSV).

Meditation

God makes himself dependent on us in order to be the means
of our rescue from the muddle and mess which the human race
has got itself into. He and the future of creation depend on
Mary's 'yes'. We depend on her allowing for his plan of
redemption to be carried out through her willingness and
co-operation.

Mary, whose word the whole world waited upon, understands even today how precariously we are teetering on the
brink of destruction. She also understands the magnitude of
responsibility entailed and the sacrifices involved in the
political decision-making of the Churches and of the world.

Every political decision has the potential for creation or
destruction. To bomb or not to bomb, to give more aid, or to

allow a few more million to starve, to support the status quo in corrupt and racist governments which benefit the few at the cost of the many, or to say 'yes' to justice and freedom from oppression.

Mary's 'yes' has set us free from the law of might. It has set us free from laws of convention which have swollen through the centuries into bigotry and fear.

Mary herself, as a young girl in Nazareth, was very much afraid of what might happen to her at the hands of convention. Single mothers were not treated kindly in those days. She understands and is with us in those fearful moments when brave decisions have to be taken. In Mary we have an intercessor who, in the way of all mothers, pleads on our behalf for God's Spirit to take possession of us more fully that we may be better held and supported in adversity and temptation and when difficult decisions have to be taken.

Action

Mary is too often a point of conflict between the denominations. Honour her today by thinking of her as the mother of the divine Christ-child who belongs to all Christians and to all the world. See yourself as a brother or sister of Christ and be united in your heart with those Christians who keep today as a very special feast.

Eleventh Sunday after Pentecost

Reading

Jesus said, 'Now the Son of Man has been glorified, and God has been glorified in him. If God has been glorified in him, God will also glorify him in himself and will glorify him at once. Little children, I am with you only a little longer. You will look for me; and as I said to the Jews so now I say to you, "where I am going, you cannot come." I give you a new commandment, that you love one another. Just as I have loved you, you also should love one another. By this everyone will know that you are my disciples, if you have love for one another' (John 13:31–6).

Meditation

We resemble Christ to the extent that we are capable of allowing love to happen through us. The glory of God is reflected in a smile. Those capable of forgetting themselves for a single second and of bestowing love in a kind word or in the smallest gesture carry the light of Christ within them and reflect it to the world, whether they consider themselves to be Christians or not.

Christian love empowers action and makes it effective, in that the least recognition of a person's fellow humanity can change that person's day, or perhaps their whole life. Love, like life itself, is energy, begetting of itself more love.

Remember what it feels like when an unknown shopkeeper or official uses a familiar or affectionate greeting – the barriers of class, money and colour melt in an instant. All at once we are kin to one another. Nothing else matters. I take with me the gift of that brief exchange which nobody can take away from me and which will warm and even fire my whole day.

In a few words of conversation with a stranger, in a smile or greeting, we meet Christ our brother.

Action

Be a channel of God's love, especially in your dealings with people who normally pass unnoticed in your life.

Be a channel of God's love to your friends as well, for our fellowship with one another is life's greatest gift. Here is a recipe for 'friendship cake' which is prepared over a ten-day period and then shared among friends. It was given to me by my next-door neighbour.

INGREDIENTS FOR STARTER

150g (5oz) plain flour
1½ tsp dried yeast or 25g (1oz) fresh yeast
1 level tsp sugar
150ml (5 fl oz) milk at blood temperature
150ml (5 fl oz) water at blood temperature

Combine the yeast, flour and sugar and add the milk and water mixture. Set aside in a warm place until frothy – about 20 minutes for fresh yeast, 30 minutes for dried, but this will always depend on room temperature.

Use a large bowl, as the mixture will rise over the 10-day period. Do not put the mixture in the fridge. Do not use an electric mixer. Use the same measuring cup throughout.

Day 1   Put the starter mixture in the bowl and add 1 cup of granulated sugar, 1 cup of plain flour, 1 cup of milk. Stir well and cover.

Day 2	Stir well
Day 3	Leave to stand
Day 4	Leave to stand
Day 5	Add 1 cup of granulated sugar, 1 cup of plain flour, 1 cup of milk. Stir well and cover.
Day 6	Stir well
Days 7, 8 & 9	Leave to stand
Day 10	Stir well. Remove 3 cups of the mixture. Keep one to start a new cake (although these cakes freeze well too) and give away the remaining two to friends.

To the remaining mixture add:

1 cup granulated sugar
2 cups plain flour
$\frac{1}{2}$ cup sultanas
$\frac{1}{2}$ cup chopped nuts, or dried fruit if you prefer
$\frac{2}{3}$ cup of sunflower oil
2 chopped cooking apples
2 eggs
2 heaped tsp baking powder
2 tsp cinnamon
2 tsp vanilla essence

Mix together and bake in a greased and lined 18cm (7 in) tin in a moderate oven (175°C, 325–350°F, Gas 3–4) for approximately $1\frac{3}{4}$ hours. Keep checking and turning the cake.

'Simone Weil'
24 August

Reading

As long as it is through obedience, I find sweetness in my deprivation of the joy of membership in the Mystical Body of Christ. For if God is willing to help me, I may thus bear witness that without this joy one can nevertheless be faithful to Christ unto death. Social enthusiasms have such power today, they raise people so effectively to the supreme degree of heroism in suffering and death, that I think it is as well that a few sheep should remain outside the fold in order to bear witness that the love of Christ is essentially something different.

> Spiritual Autobiography: *Waiting On God*
> Simone Weil

Meditation

If Simone Weil were to be officially canonised, she might be called the patron saint of all misfits and rebels! Real holiness often begins outside the institutional Church, for God works in mysterious ways through the most unlikely people. The Christian faith is not an elitist club; or, if it is, its members are so well camouflaged in God's love that they are only recognised by what they leave behind.

Sometimes it is important not to be identified as 'Christians' at all, so that the love of Christ can quietly enfold someone without anyone taking the credit for it except God's Spirit, to whom the credit belongs. It is often in our own doubts and confusion that the faith of another person takes root. He or she is given confidence in Christ by the ability of Christians to be comfortable in their ordinary humanity. All the greatest saints and teachers of spirituality have been communicators and unafraid of the world's noticing their weaknesses or the flaws in their personality.

Christ himself became a human being in order to share in our humanity and in the consequence of human beings out of tune with God. The honesty of people who acknowledge their own disconnectedness with God, which may be due in part to disillusion concerning the manifest nature of the institutional Church or Christians known to them, gives heart to those who might not feel 'good enough' to know God intimately.

Christ set aside the majesty and glory of the Godhead in order to reach out to us in the sharing of our human nature, so we too must abandon any smug feeling of having 'arrived' in our spirituality. Only then shall we be able to reach out to our brothers and sisters with empathy and love. The rest is worked on their hearts in ways beyond our understanding.

Action

If you have a friend who is in any way a rebel, or who does not quite fit into your social circle, invite them for a meal and by your behaviour towards them make them feel welcome and cherished in your house.

Twelfth Sunday after Pentecost

Reading

I do not pray for these only, but also for those who believe in me through their word, that they may all be one; even as thou, Father, art in me, and I in thee, that they also may be in us, so that the world may believe that thou hast sent me. The glory which thou hast given me I have given to them, that they may be one even as we are one, I in them and thou in me, that they may bcome perfectly one, so that the world may know that thou hast sent me and hast loved them even as thou hast loved me. Father, I desire that they also, whom thou hast given me, may be with me where I am, to behold my glory which thou hast given me, in thy love for me before the foundation of the world. O righteous Father, the world has not known thee, but I have known thee; and these know that thou hast sent me. I made known to them thy name, and I will make it known, that the love with which thou hast loved me may be in them, and I in them (John 17:20–end).

Meditation

We are one but we are not homogeneous. Our kinship in Christ does not bear the slightest trace of uniformity, for the separate existence of every person on earth is bound up in God as the petals of a flower together form a single bloom. We know his love through the secret centre of our inner being because we have Christ's Spirit living in us. The kingdom of heaven is the abiding presence of the living God in each person on earth.

God loves the whole person beginning from the heart, which is the essence of a human being, that true centre where we have our beginning. The things which are added or taken from us in life only surround this centre. It is not in them, but through them that God's love is fully consummated. Nothing we do can either add or take away from it because God's love is complete and perfect, as God is complete and perfect and has been since before all ages.

The heart of the individual who knows God is the heart of Christ himself and all the separate human beings on earth who recognise and respond to the love of God through the means given to them are the body of Christ, what we call the Church on earth.

The living Christ is in us and in all that is good in creation and we are one with him in the love of the Father.

Be conscious of belonging. Know and be grateful for the bonds of family, community and society. Be conscious of belonging to the earth, the sea, the sky and trees – even the weather.

Action

Go for a walk today. If you find yourself in a group, at work or at a party, be conscious of belonging to the wider world and fully enjoy that moment.

Saint Augustine of Hippo
28 August

Reading

*My soul, you too must listen to the word of God. Do not be
foolish; do not let the din of your folly deafen the ears of your
heart. For the Word himself calls you to return. In him is the
place of peace that cannot be disturbed, and he will not withold
himself from your love unless you withold your love from him.*

The Confessions of Saint Augustine, Book 4

Meditation

All matter was loved into existence by a God who made all
things essentially good. Life itself was spoken into being out of
silence. All the material things with which we are surrounded
and driven are chaotic noise which penetrates into the essence
of a human being. The Creator God spoke perfect harmony
out of chaos and void. To pay attention to noise is to ignore
the call of the Creator to life.

At the heart of the world's noise the Incarnate Word of God
whispers an invitation to us to meet him in our own place of
inner silence. He himself came to us in the silence of anony-
mity and poverty, so we must meet him in the silence of our
own nothingness, of accepting who and what we are and of
desiring him in that situation.

If the distractions and pressures of life have drawn us a long
way from this place of silence, we are called to return, to effect
a *metanoia,* or repentance in ourselves. In returning to the
essence of who and what we are, and in accepting and loving

that person, we find peace and fulfilment, wisdom and understanding and the Christ-child at the heart of it all.

Action

Modelling with clay is a good way to experience matter and of
bringing coherence out of what is formless, so if you can get
hold of some clay, try this as an experiment.

Enjoy the feel of the clay and enjoy playing with it. All
creative work is play. Play with the material and let it shape
itself into being under the guidance of your hand while you let
the ideas in the meditation take the form they are meant to
take for you in your mind and heart.

A practical point: clay should be kept moist at all times, so
when you have finished with it, wrap it in wet cloth and put a
damp rag over the piece you are working on, so that you can
continue tomorrow. If it is still too hard to work easily,
sprinkle it liberally with water.

Thirteenth Sunday after Pentecost

Reading

Now a Jew named Apollos, a native of Alexandria, came to Ephesus. He was an eloquent man, well versed in the scriptures. He had been instructed in the way of the Lord; and being fervent in spirit, he spoke and taught accurately the things concerning Jesus, though he knew only the baptism of John. He began to speak boldly in the synagogue; but when Priscilla and Aquila heard him, they took him and expounded to him the way of God more accurately. And when he wished to cross to Achaia, the brethren encouraged him, and wrote to the disciples to receive him. When he arrived, he greatly helped those who through grace had believed, for he powerfully confuted the Jews in public, showing by the scriptures that the Christ was Jesus (Acts 18:24–end).

Meditation

The hand of God is invariably gentle, for it is the women of the company who take the enthusiastic, if somewhat naïve disciple to one side, in order to 'expound to him the way of God more accurately.' The descendants of this well-meaning disciple are very much with us today. We meet them in the street, distributing leaflets and strumming guitars. They are full of love for God and the very best of intentions, but it is quite likely that the number of people they put off the Christian faith far exceeds those they convert – and all for lack of instruction.

We are called in the service of Christ to engage all of our faculties and to give of all of the talents and resources at our disposal. It is therefore of the utmost importance that the intellect of every Christian disciple, no matter how limited, be sharpened and exercised to the full. There is a great need for the Priscillas and Aquilas of the world to come forward and lay on our hearts the gentle touch of wisdom and learning. A charismatic personality, in other words the ability to attract people and to excite their interest, is of very little use if the people whose interest they have aroused are left without any kind of intellectual challenge. We are called to respond to the needs of an increasingly educated world where people are crying out to be fed intellectually as well as emotionally, as we are called to build one another up to the full stature of maturity.

Desire true wisdom and right judgment in matters of faith. Be with Priscilla and Aquila and include in your company anyone known to you who is actively involved in the work of evangelism.

Action

Try to broaden your understanding of other people's faith, and to deepen your own, by reading and learning as much as possible. Your local priest or pastor is an excellent person to turn to for advice, as his or her training will have involved a considerable amount of formal study. It is a great pity that these valuable resources (which usually include a thorough grounding in Greek and Hebrew) are so often neglected by the average parishioner, especially as most vicars will be only too happy to share the learning which they have acquired with anyone who is interested. There are also a number of courses, leading to a certificate or diploma in theology, which are extremely interesting and well worth doing. Again, ask your vicar, and if you really don't think you have the intellect or time for formal study ask him to point you to a few helpful books.

If you are lucky enough to have plenty of books of your own on theology or spirituality that you can spare for a while, why not start a small lending library at the back of your church?

Fourteenth Sunday after Pentecost

Reading

Each of you, however, should love his wife as himself, and a wife should respect her husband.

Children, obey your parents in the Lord, for this is right. 'Honour your father and mother' – this is the first commandment with a promise: 'so that it may be well with you and you may live long on the earth.'

And, fathers, do not provoke your children to anger, but bring them up in the discipline and instruction of the Lord (Eph. 5:33–6:4).

Meditation

The family has been called a school for charity; not pious insipid charity, but full-bodied and courageous human love. The family is God's gift to humanity, supplying the need of human beings to belong to one another and to belong to a community or nation.

Christ himself needed to belong to family and community and in his own experience of loneliness in the wilderness, in the garden at Gethsemane, in great crowds and when he was misunderstood by friends and by religious officials, he identified with all those who in some way do not belong. The Son of Man himself 'has nowhere to lay his head'.

Christ is present to all loneliness. He is in the loneliness of a marriage or relationship where two people have long since lost touch with one another and gone after material things or success. He weeps with those who have been deprived of land and nationality and he is present to the loneliness of success. Christ fully knows the sadness of the one who is so 'international' that he or she no longer knows where or to whom they belong. The loneliness of the rich and the multi-national is the most pathetic poverty.

Christ speaks to the heart of individuals when they acknowledge their need to belong through him to the family of humanity. The Cross of Christ is our bridge, the means whereby we link up with one another in the cold desert of modern life and reaffirm our membership of the human family in the unspoken bond of the heart.

Action

Strengthen family ties by writing a letter to a relative you have lost touch with or by responding in some way to an appeal from your local community or church. It does not have to involve giving money. Time and commitment are more costly than the signing of a cheque. If you can identify with one of the many charities trying to alleviate suffering and poverty in the world, give them some of your time and resources.

Holy Cross Day
14 September

Reading

For the message about the cross is foolishness to those who are perishing, but to us who are being saved it is the power of God. For it is written, 'I will destroy the wisdom of the wise, and the discernment of the discerning I will thwart.' Where is the one who is wise? Where is the scribe? Where is the debater of this age? Has not God made foolish the wisdom of the world? For since, in the wisdom of God, the world did not know God through wisdom, God decided, through the foolishness of our proclamation, to save those who believe. For Jews demand signs and Greeks desire wisdom, but we proclaim Christ crucified, a stumbling block to Jews and foolishness to Gentiles, but to those who are the called, both Jews and Greeks, Christ the power of God and the wisdom of God. For God's foolishness is wiser than human wisdom, and God's weakness is stronger than human strength (1 Cor. 1:18–25).

Meditation

The Cross is worn as jewellery in order to disguise its foolishness. The manner of Christ's death was a scandal, even in its day, and we have overlaid it with gold to cover up the scandal so that it can be more easily absorbed into our value system. There was nothing beautiful about the manner in which Jesus was tortured and put to death. There is nothing beautiful about raw suffering. It does not ennoble people. It demeans them. So in identifying in any way with the Cross of

Christ, we are at best eccentric and, in the eyes of most, embarrassing and silly.

There is nothing noble about admitting to a living faith, but Christ endured the ignoble to its utmost limits so that we need never be ashamed of representing him to the world, even without saying anything. The eccentricity and silliness of admitting to the centrality of the Cross and to the power of the risen Christ in one's life are utter foolishness and at the same time wisdom itself.

Wisdom is given to the 'foolish' because their vision has not become clouded by cleverness. How many people in the world who have never given themselves over to a moment's spiritual foolishness end up as alcoholics or chronic depressives, full of a sense of failure and bitterness?

Wisdom is the bedrock of our existence. It has nothing to do with cleverness or intelligence. It is simply a rock on which our feet are firmly planted in a world of shifting values and shallow friendships. A wise person inspires confidence in others. Foolish and total love for God and for other human beings is neither clever or practical. It contributes nothing useful to modern life and yet today more than ever, the foolish wisdom of reconciliation, the bringing together of the whole of creation in the Cross of Christ, is essential for our happiness and survival.

Action

The most beautiful cross I ever owned was made for me by my ten-year-old daughter out of papier mâché. Here is how she made it:

Bind together two matches with cotton to form a cross. Cut some newspaper into strips. Make a paste of flour and water and stick the newspaper all over the cross using the paste. Put the cross in a very slow oven to dry for 3 or 4 hours. You can then paint, glaze or wax the finished cross once it has cooled.

Fifteenth Sunday after Pentecost

Reading

The Lord is gracious and merciful,
*   slow to anger and abounding in steadfast love.*
The Lord is good to all,
*   and his compassion is over all that he has made.*
All your works shall give thanks to you, O Lord,
*   and all your faithful shall bless you.*
They shall speak of the glory of your kingdom,
*   and tell of your power,*
to make known to all people your mighty deeds,
*   and the glorious splendour of your kingdom.*
Your kingdom is an everlasting kingdom,
*   and your dominion endures throughout all generation*
                                             (Ps. 145:8–13).

Meditation

There was a brief spell during the Gulf War of 1990 when both
sides of the House of Commons seemed to be in harmony with
each other, working together to find the solution to a crisis in
the best interests of the nation and of everyone concerned.
Gone was the usual bar-room brawl atmosphere and even
with the limited view afforded by television coverage, it was
clear that the 'dominion' which was in power far outshone the
tawdriness of party politics.

Our human existence is bound up in a higher order. Perhaps
we ourselves are bound individually to the angels and superior

beings who belong to that order (I personally believe in guardian angels) as we are bound to one another in relationships and as a global family. The decisions taken by our governments affect us as individuals and how we lead our lives in the context of those decisions affects millions of human beings, plants and animals in other parts of the world. What I consume and what I throw away affect the environment and the societies whose customs and needs are different from mine.

Our worldly order corresponds to something divine and eternal. It is reaching out to that eternal order and growing closer to it day by day and minute by minute, wherever there is peace and reconciliation between nations or political parties, or between the interests of the consumer against those of the environment and of people living in the third world. The spirit of the Creator God, his compassion for the world, hovers over us and our human predicament, as it hovered over the darkness and void before the beginning of the world.

Go over the reading again, savouring each phrase. If you feel that any of it touches you in a particular way, stay with it and come back to it later on in the day if you feel like it, or keep it with you in the silence of your inner being as you go about the work of the coming week.

Action

Be a means for reconciliation. More and more materials are capable of being recycled which gives us all something positive to do in the interest of conservation and makes us able to contribute directly to the well-being of others by cutting down on waste. If there is somewhere near you where newspapers, aluminium, cardboard, etc., can be recycled, plan to make a habit of using these facilities. Recognise and affirm our bond with people from poorer nations by buying their products, especially those produced by co-operatives which are run by the people themselves.

Saint Matthew, Apostle and Evangelist
21 September

Reading

As Jesus was walking along, he saw a man called Matthew sitting at the tax booth; and he said to him, 'Follow me.' And he got up and followed him. And as he sat at dinner in the house, many tax collectors and sinners came and were sitting with him and disciples. When the Pharisees saw this, they said to his disciples, 'Why does your teacher eat with tax collectors and sinners?' But when he heard this, he said, 'Those who are well have no need of a physician, but those who are sick. Go and learn what this means, "I desire mercy, not sacrifice." For I have come to call not the righteous but sinners' (Matt. 9:9–13 NRSV)

Meditation

Matthew was called to preach the good news. The Greek word, *euangelos* means good news, and the good news lives on: that Christ the Son of God has not come to sit comfortably with the acceptable and virtuous, but has taken his place among the miscreants and misfits of society.

Rightness with God and rightness with one another and with the created world mean penetrating the invisible shield which surrounds separate human beings, and which divides families and nations. Forgiveness and reconciliation involve, first of all, a breaking-down of shields and barriers.

This century has seen a great deal of breaking-down of barriers and of Christ eating and drinking in our midst as he raises up the people and situations which hitherto seemed hopeless. The first men and women to cross the broken wall in Berlin, to be reconciled with their families and friends and with the other half of their nation, met Christ as they climbed over the rubble of years of hatred and oppression. The good news is that Christ is the means for breaking down the barriers of prejudice, mistrust and the legacy of conflict inherited from previous generations. He is present at the heart of the unthinkable, eating and drinking with what is hopeless and rejected in the individual and between nations.

It is therefore imperative that we, as his disciples, make it our life's work to break down the barriers that exist between us and between us and our world, that we 'eat and drink' with one another, with Christ in our midst, at every possible opportunity.

Action

Do something towards breaking down a barrier, either in a relationship, or on a more global scale. If there is prejudice in the conversation around you, seek to stabilise the negative feelings and try to prevent the person articulating them from becoming isolated.

Presents are a good way of breaking down barriers, especially if they are made by the giver, so try making or giving something of your own. Here is a recipe for home-made fudge which goes down extremely well with almost anybody:

EQUIPMENT

1 large heavy-based saucepan

1 metal tablespoon
1 sugar thermometer
1 wooden spoon
1 lightly greased shallow tin 20cm × 15cm (8in 6in)
1 sharp knife

INGREDIENTS

450g (1lb) granulated sugar
50g (2oz) butter
5 fl oz (14 pint) evaporated milk
5 fl.oz. (14 pint) fresh milk
3 drops vanilla essence

1   Put the sugar, butter and both sorts of milk into the
saucepan and heat very gently, stirring with the tablespoon
until all the sugar has dissolved and the fat has melted. Bring
the mixture to the boil and boil steadily until the thermometer
registers 116°C/240°F. Stir the mixture occasionally.
2   Remove the pan from the heat and place on a cold surface,
such as a stainless steel top.
3   Add the vanilla essence and beat the mixture with the
wooden spoon until it becomes thick and creamy and slightly
granular.
4   Pour the fudge into the greased tin immediately, otherwise
it will set in the pan. Leave until nearly cold.
5   Cut the cooled fudge into squares with the sharp knife
and put them in a decorated box which you can make
yourself.

Here is how to make a simple box large enough to take ½ lb of
fudge:
    Draw the diagram overleaf on plain or coloured card
following the dimensions given. Make sure the measurements
are accurate and that the corners are 90 degrees.

Cut out along the solid lines. If the card is fairly thick score it along the out side. If you are using lightweight card, fold along the dotted lines or, better still, fold each dotted line in turn against the edge of a ruler.

Glue A to B and leave to dry. Fold in the remaining tabs and the lid and base at top and bottom.

Paint or decorate the box or leave it plain and tie with a bow.

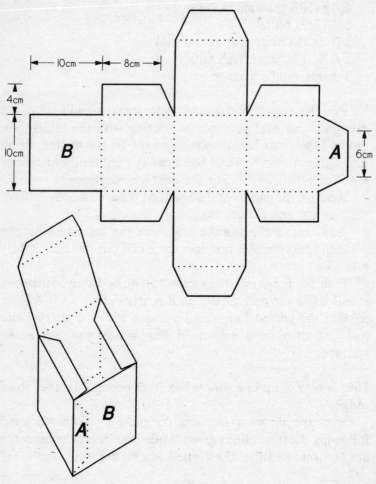

Sixteenth Sunday after Pentecost

Reading

Do not be overcome by evil, but overcome evil with good (Rom. 12:21).

Meditation

Christ's Passion begins where heroism ends. Hatred is overcome by quiet love, a sort of gentle Gulf Stream that warms the coldness surrounding the person who suffers at the hands of another. Its unseen presence brings about imperceptible change in the evil of that situation because the difference would only be felt if the warm current were to be suddenly cut off.

Evil is confronted in the commonplace because it manifests itself most often in the ordinary. Hatred is overcome by an allowing of love to pour into the victim of hatred so that it can flow on through that person to its perpetrator. Christ, the ultimate good, allowed himself to be poured out in this way on to the world's evil, or sin.

The sin of the world lies in its failing to harmonise with the ultimate good which is love itself. The world's pain and confusion, its sickness and fear are part of the noise that has come of the interference with the music of God's love. If a radio is badly tuned it will eventually give the listener a headache and if the bad tuning was all that could be heard for a year it would undoubtedly lead to madness. The world has allowed itself to be mistuned for thousands of years. All

297

the world's pain and suffering are caught up in the cacophany of its bad tuning, but when hatred is met with compassion, harmony supersedes the crackle, as when the aerial in a car is able to pick up the programme it had lost while driving under a tunnel.

Every kind of sin is ministered to by allowing Christ to reorientate the radio so that it can pick up the sound waves. When the person who most hurts me opens up old wounds, even if he or she does so unwittingly, it is Christ in me who creates a bridge between us and the possibility for harmony. When my enemy slanders and vilifies me and steals my friends, it is Christ whom I meet and with whom I confront the lies and all the pain which that person has wittingly or unwittingly caused me in the past.

I achieve nothing by speaking for myself, or by requiting the deeds of my oppressor, because I do not see the situation as Christ sees it from the vantage point of the Cross. I therefore tentatively allow the music of the love of God to flow into that situation, knowing that he sees and understands all and has already begun the process of reconciliation.

Action

Next time you are listening to the car radio and you lose touch with the programme, so that the sound becomes very crackly or faint, hold the world and all those who do not hear or feel the love of God in their lives into a moment of centring. If you know of an individual to whom this applies, concentrate especially on that person.

Saint Michael and All Angels
29 September

Reading

O ye Angels of the Lord, bless ye the Lord: praise him, and magnify him for ever.

The Book of Common Prayer in Wales

Meditation

Angels are messengers (the Greek word *angellos* means messenger) and their presence is often manifested in the message itself. A novel or magazine article can embody a truth or bring comfort in a way which is quite unrelated to the general sense of the text. The same is true with radio or television. A sudden and immediate experience of goodness or happiness, or of being loved comes while watching a film or listening to the radio. Sometimes new hope for the future is suddenly present where it had not been before, or we feel reassured in the taking of a decision. It is quite likely that none of these things had any relevance to the film itself. It is equally likely that 'coincidence' has led us to a play or a novel which is of immediate relevance to our situation.

Angels are everywhere, not as insipid creatures in diaphanous nightshirts, but as supernatural beings, hidden in the elemental forces of fire and wind, of rain and snow. They are the retinue of the Spirit of God. When the eyes of the servant of Elisha were opened he saw the army of God's angels encamped around the Israelites, to protect them from the King of Syria (see 2 Kgs. 6:8–18).

If the eyes of our hearts were opened we too would see the reality of God's angels surrounding us on every side, as heaven itself surrounds the world we live in.

Action

Here is a recipe for angel cake. You will need a 22cm (9in) non-stick cake tin.

INGREDIENTS

   75g (6oz) castor sugar
   100/125g (4oz) self-raising flour
   ½ tsp salt
   10–12 egg whites
   1 tsp cream of tartar
   ½ tsp vanilla essence

Preheat oven to 180°C (350°F, Gas 4).

Sift the sugar thoroughly.

Sift the flour 3 times with 50g (2oz) of the sifted sugar and the salt. It is essential that the sugar and flour be completely lump-free if the cake is to attain its ultimate angelic lightness.

Whip the egg whites until stiff but not dry and add the cream of tartar.

Gradually whip in about 1 tablespoon at a time a further 50g (2oz) of the sifted sugar.

Fold the vanilla essence into the mixture by hand. Sift the remaining sugar and the flour on to the batter and fold it in gently by hand, using a rubber or wooden scraper.

Pour the batter into the greased cake tin and bake for about 40 minutes. Invert the cake and allow it to cool and set.

Be sure to remove the cake from the tin before storing it in an air-tight container.

When ready to eat, the cake should be gently prised apart with two forks, rather than cut with a knife.

HARVEST-TIDE

Harvest Festival

Reading

The one who sows sparingly will also reap sparingly, and the one who sows bountifully will also reap bountifully. Each of you must give as you have made up your mind, not reluctantly or under compulsion, for God loves a cheerful giver. And God is able to provide you with every blessing in abundance, so that by always having enough of everything, you may share abundantly in every good work. As it is written, 'He scatters abroad, he gives to the poor; his righteousness endures forever.' He who supplies seed to the sower and bread for food will supply and multiply your seed for sowing and increase the harvest of your right-eousness. You will be enriched in every way for your great generosity, which will produce thanksgiving to God through us (2 Cor. 9:6–11).

Meditation

Life itself is the fruit of the harvest. It is to be lived with generosity and abandon. It is to be entered into recklessly, as one enters into the sea on a hot day, confident of the cooling water, exhilarated by the waves, forgetful for a moment of weighty and sensible things. Fun is of the Holy Spirit. It is never shallow or vulgar, but profound and unquenchable, like the sort of birthday candles which rekindle themselves after they have been blown out.

We reap what we sow, so that if laughter and fun overflow from our reciprocal love for God, we pass these things on to others, for we are the harvest and at the same time the means whereby the world is harvested into the love of God. Life is not to be lived meanly, for joy and love are spread by human beings living fully as they are created to be, in a wholehearted allowing of themselves to be known by the Lord of the harvest.

In allowing the harvest of ourselves to be sown and reaped in us, all whom we meet are blessed. They receive in abundance, for nothing is ours to hold. Everything is lent for a while, so that when today's riches are required of us others may be given in their place, that the harvest of our righteousness may be increased.

Action

Don't quench the Holy Spirit by stifling fun. Allow a little frivolity into your life in first inviting and allowing God's Holy Spirit to blow in whatever way throughout your whole day. Don't think consciously about what effect this is having on others, but be fully yourself, fully engaged in the business of living.

This is the season for harvesting apples. Toffee apples are most children's (and some adults') idea of fun, so make a batch this week.

EQUIPMENT

1 large heavy-based saucepan
1 sugar thermometer
6 thin wooden or paper lollipop sticks
1 greased baking tray

INGREDIENTS

6 Granny Smith apples (or any fairly sour eating apple)
450g (1lb) demerara sugar
50g (2oz) butter
2 tsp vinegar
150ml ($\frac{1}{4}$pt) water
6 tbsp golden syrup

Put the sugar, butter, vinegar, water and golden syrup into the saucepan.

Heat the ingredients gently until the sugar dissolves, then boil rapidly until the temperature reaches 145°C. (290°F).

While the syrup is coming to the correct temperature, wipe the apples and push the sticks into the cores.

Dip the apples quickly into the toffee, twirling them round for a few seconds and stand them on the greased baking tray until set.

Seventeenth Sunday after Pentecost

Reading

After he had ended all his sayings in the hearing of the people he entered Capernaum. Now a centurion had a slave who was dear to him, who was sick and at the point of death. When he heard of Jesus, he sent to him elders of the Jews, asking him to come and heal his slave. And when they came to Jesus, they besought him earnestly, saying, 'He is worthy to have you do this for him, for he loves our nation, and he built us our synagogue.' And Jesus went with them. When he was not far from the house, the centurion sent friends to him, saying to him, 'Lord, do not trouble yourself, for I am not worthy to have you come under my roof; therefore I did not presume to come to you. But say the word, and let my servant be healed. For I am a man set under authority, with soldiers under me: and I say to one, "Go" and he goes; and to another, "Come", and he comes; and to my slave, "Do this", and he does it'. When Jesus heard this he marvelled at him, and turned and said to the multitude that followed him, 'I tell you, not even in Israel have I found such faith.' And when those who had been sent returned to the house, they found the slave well (Luke 7:1–10).

Meditation

Bring someone known to you into this situation. Let it be a person who is in need of some form of healing, either physical or spiritual. It could be a colleague at work, a friend or relative, or someone on whom you depend for practical help.

First embrace that person in your own heart and affirm your love for them. If they are suffering in some way, hold their pain close to you and allow it into God's love on their behalf. Seek Jesus, perhaps with some difficulty, going from place to place until you find him. You can search for him in your own surroundings or in a place of your imagination. Either way, let the scene present itself to you of its own accord. Don't impose and don't strain.

When you have found the Lord, tell him about your friend. You can do this with words, but if words seem inadequate or superfluous, simply allow him into the love you have for that person. Stay with this moment or come back to it when distractions draw you aside. Note what Jesus says to you and to others around you and anything he might say concerning your friend. Don't worry if nothing gets said. The holding of that person in the love of Christ is enough.

Do this meditation a couple of times, if possible, starting from the point where you felt the presence of the Lord most keenly.

Action

If you have been praying for a particular person during this meditation, visit them or write to them.

Feast of the Guardian Angels
2 October

Reading

Behold, I send an angel before you, to guard you on the way and to bring you to the place which I have prepared. Give heed to him and hearken to his voice, do not rebel against him, for he will not pardon your transgression; for my name is in him. But if you hearken attentively to his voice and do all that I say, then I will be an enemy to your enemies and an adversary to your adversaries (Exod. 23:20–2).

Meditation

At the time of the Mau-Mau uprising in Kenya in the early 1950s, a group of English missionaries were surrounded one night by people who had come to burn down the mission house and kill its occupants. However, the attack was aborted at the last minute because, according to later reports, the attackers saw that the house was surrounded by heavily armed men who greatly outnumbered them.

One day my sister's little girl, who was then less than two years old, wandered out of the front door of their house in London which had inadvertently been left open by one of the other children. Just as they were all getting ready to call the police the child reappeared between two strangers. Young men in their early twenties, they had escorted her home, having found her in the middle of the road at some distance from the house.

We are not alone. We live in the company of angels. They

are masters of disguise and camouflage, emissaries of God's Holy Spirit, manifestations of the imminence of heaven, who guard us from danger and the powers and principalities of darkness. In stillness and purity of heart and in vulnerability to love it is just possible to catch a glimpse of them in a seeming reflection, a passing shadow, in the stranger who appears in a crisis, in the single word of comfort spoken from an unlikely source. Angels are messengers from heaven disguised in the message they bring.

Action

Read some of the fairy scenes in Shakespeare's *Midsummer Night's Dream* for a different perspective in angels. Be open to the idea that heaven – and angels – may be closer than we realise.

Saint Francis of Assisi
4 October

Reading

Lord make me
An instrument of thy peace;
Where there is hate that I may bring love,
Where there is offence that I may bring pardon,
Where there is discord that I may bring union,
Where there is error that I may bring truth,
Where there is doubt that I may bring faith,
Where there is despair that I may bring hope,
Where there is darkness that I may bring light,
Where there is sadness that I may bring joy.

O Master, make me
Not so much to be consoled as to console;
Not so much to be loved as to love;
Not so much to be understood as to understand;
For it is in giving that one receives;
It is in self-forgetfulness that one finds;
It is in pardoning that one is pardoned;
It is in dying that one finds eternal life.

Prayer of St Francis of Assisi

Meditation

To be a human being, made in the image and likeness of God
is a great privilege. To be in the position of reflecting into the
world the love which loved us into existence and which bought

us back from ultimate destruction is an honour. It is an honour which is crowned and affirmed in our being permitted to be co-creators with him and participators in the on-going process of the world's redemption which was begun and continues in Christ.

We are the means whereby God works in the world. The miracle of his coming to us and of his continual presence lies in his setting aside of his omnipotence to make himself needful of us. We have a choice – to respond to his need or to ignore it with indifference.

Pray about this reading as you did the one on the fifteenth Sunday after Pentecost, page 289.

Action

Apply any one of the means of being an instrument of God's peace described in the prayer of St Francis to a situation which you know. Begin by bringing that person or situation into your time of stillness in God and allow for his Holy spirit to indicate what specific course of action you should take.

Eighteenth Sunday after Pentecost

Reading

The end of all things is near; therefore be serious and discipline yourselves for the sake of your prayers. Above all, maintain constant love for one another, for love covers a multitude of sins. Be hospitable to one another without complaining. Like good stewards of the manifold grace of God, serve one another with whatever gift each of you has received. Whoever speaks must do so as one speaking the very words of God; whoever serves must do so with the strength that God supplies, so that God may be glorified in all things through Jesus Christ. To him belong the glory and the power forever and ever. Amen (1Pet. 4:7–11 NRSV).

Meditation

Nothing we have can really be said to belong to us. Talents and material assets are on loan. They are placed in our hands in order that we might be happy. God wants, above all, that human beings should be happy and, since a human being is created in love in the image and likeness of the God of love, it follows that happiness can only be attained by being continually receptive to the action of God's love for the one he has created. A gift or talent which is not permanently vulnerable to being imbued with the love of God and with his life-giving Spirit turns in on itself and ultimately shrivels up and dies.

Our work is our prayer. Writers and artists live in fear of 'blocks' and of being 'burnt out' creatively but perfect love casts out this kind of fear. If a writer or painter waits on God and is vulnerable to the touch of his Spirit, his or her work will flower and bear fruit in the fullness of time. The same is true for all other professions.

Blocks and burnt-out periods exist for everyone in one form or another. They can be caused by overtiredness, stress or anxiety. They can also be caused by people neglecting the source of their talent, whether the talent consists in being a good parent, a good cook, or a competent store manager or leader of a community. All talent comes of the love of God and depends on that love for its continuing growth and all work needs to be orientated to that source.

Take some time to look at where you stand regarding your chosen profession or call in life. If the fire that was in your original call seems to be burning rather low at the moment, let that feeling be vulnerable to the action of the fire of God's creator Spirit.

Action

If you have any control or influence in the working life of another person (a colleague or employee) do what you can to support them and develop their talents.

Let your work, whatever it is, be brought into the presence of Christ. See yourself in your job with Christ there beside you. Note any feelings of fulfilment and happiness or boredom and frustration.

Hold in your time of silence with God any person known to you who is experiencing difficulties at work.

Nineteenth Sunday after Pentecost

Reading

Faith is the assurance of things hoped for, the conviction of things not seen (Heb. 11:1).

Meditation

Faith transcends belief. Believing in something, whether it is in Father Christmas or in the loyalty of a friend, does not have the endurance of faith. The thing believed in may or may not fail the test of time. Faith in God comes of conviction. It comes of having seen and known, of having experienced God for ourselves.

There is a sense in which faith can never be taken from us, because it is as irrefutable as an event which has already happened, except that it is not fixed in the past. The living faith given to us by the action of God's Holy Spirit is continually growing and adapting itself to the present.

Faith is a garment which grows with a person as protection from the bad weather of every kind of adversity. A person's knowledge and experience of God are fixed in the present moment and yet are as fluid as water, as free as air.

Faith is far more than looking forward to something in the future – heaven, perhaps or 'salvation'. It is hope realised in the present. The kingdom of heaven is here and now in our very midst – on the station platform, in the supermarket, at the airport, in all the anonymous places where people congregate

and in the secret heart of every person. It waits to be acknowl-
edged, to be realised.

Faith is the presence of the Holy Spirit waiting to recognise
and be recognised in the eyes of another person. It is like a
candle needing to be lit from the flame of another person's
smile, or word of encouragement, or genuine affection. Faith
is blocked whenever love is held back.

Action

Light a nightlight which burns for eight hours, as a symbol of
enduring faith and of the presence of the Holy Spirit in your
home and in your heart. Better still, if you can persuade your
priest to let you have some of the oil used for the sacristy lamp,
have a permanent light burning somewhere in your house.
Make sure you have a smoke alarm, though.

Affirm these actions by allowing the flame of the love of
God to light others by your treatment of them.

Saint Luke
18 October

Reading

The seventy returned with joy, saying, 'Lord, in your name even the demons submit to us!' he said to them, 'I watched Satan fall from heaven like a flash of lightning. See, I have given you authority to tread on snakes and scorpions, and over all the power of the enemy; and nothing will hurt you. Nevertheless, do not rejoice at this, that the spirits submit to you, but rejoice that your names are written in heaven' (Luke 10:17–20).

Gospel for the Orthodox Liturgy

Meditation

There is a freshness and innocence about the early Church which has become clouded with the passage of time. Rarely, even in the most charismatic circles, does worship have that blend of innocence, untroubled joy and the sense of the imminence of Emmanuel, God with us. As Christians we need to dare to feel thrilled by the power of the risen Christ in our lives and in the world.

Experience this moment with the seventy who had returned with joy. They are like excited children returning to a much-loved older brother, even to a mother, for Christ is all things to all people. We too should be excited by each new discovery pertaining to our faith and by every new door which is opened to us on our journey towards God and towards overcoming the difficulties which we face in our search for him.

Saint Luke was a doctor, so now is a good time to be

thankful for all doctors, nurses and medical personnel, as well as for hospitals, day care centres and our local surgeries. Bring them, and especially any known to you, into your time of silence with God, in order that they too may feel his healing touch.

Action

Allow yourself to feel genuine excitement and pleasure over something you have accomplished or seen someone else accomplish. If you normally keep these things to yourself, share the good news with a friend.

Last Sunday after Pentecost
Nineteenth Sunday after Trinity

Reading

I consider that the sufferings of this present time are not worth comparing with the glory about to be revealed to us. For the creation waits with eager longing for the revealing of the children of God ... We know that the whole creation has been groaning in labour pains until now; and not only the creation, but we ourselves, who have the first fruits of the Spirit, groan inwardly while we wait for adoption, the redemption of our bodies. For in hope we were saved. Now hope that is seen is not hope. For who hopes for what is seen? But if we hope for what we do not see, we wait for it with patience (Rom. 8:18–19, 22–5).

Meditation

It is said that some species of plant can be heard to grow. Their expanding tissue and multiplying cells creak as they stretch and the sound can be speeded up and amplified. Growth is always painful because it involves so much dying and so much leaving behind of the things of the past.

Growth and suffering are bound up in each other. We groan and creak as we grow and suffer and wait; wait for circumstances to improve, for the healing of sickness, for a turn in material fortunes and for the earth itself to be healed of all the sickness to which it has been subjected by the greed and selfishness of humanity. Waiting, especially long-term waiting, is the most enervating experience.

But we have in our midst the source of life and energy, the

wind and fire of God's Holy Spirit who transforms our waiting into vitality. Life is a time of waiting on God, the Lord of laughter and hope and of the great Dance of creation. The isolation of people in a time of waiting for their own individual salvation to be worked out is already rewarded in Christ's identifying with our loneliness and with the apparent futility of suffering.

He is forsaken and forgotten with us on Calvary, ignored and rejected at Bethlehem, but waits for us in the risen Christ by the shore of the Galilean sea, at the supper in Emmaus and at the very heart of our separation and darkness.

Action

Understand from the heart what long-term waiting feels like for a young person who is paralysed for life after an accident, for a hostage or prisoner serving a life sentence, for those still seeking relatives lost in the Second World War. If you know of anyone in this kind of situation, give them time and empathy.

Support the work of organisations which try to help prisoners, such as Amnesty International or the Prison Phoenix Trust.

Twentieth Sunday after Trinity
Ninth before Christmas

Reading

Then Jesus told them a parable about their need to pray always and not to lose heart. He said, 'In a certain city there was a judge who neither feared God nor had respect for people. In that city there was a widow who kept coming to him and saying, "Grant me justice against my opponent." For a while he refused; but later he said to himself, "Though I have no fear of God and no respect for anyone, yet because this widow keeps bothering me, I will grant her justice, so that she may not wear me out by continually coming."' And the Lord said, 'Listen to what the unjust judge says. And will not God grant justice to his chosen ones who cry to him day and night? Will he delay long in helping them? I tell you, he will quickly grant justice to them. And yet, when the Son of Man comes, will he find faith on earth?' (Luke 18:1–8 NRSV).

Meditation

Prayer begins with openness to the possibility of God being manifested in the circumstances of daily life, or in a sudden acute awareness of a super-human love which seems to come from nowhere. It is also about responding to that experience and being prepared for it to happen. God comes quietly. It is not his way to shock and frighten those he loves. When the Son of Man comes then, will he find anyone prepared to receive the experience of God?

The Son of Man is to be trusted in his coming. He never

trambles on dreams, even inadvertently, neither does he put people down or humiliate them in any way. But sometimes his presence is not clearly felt, as though he had temporarily left on some errand, like a parent who goes to answer the telephone, leaving the young child in the room next door. The child's horizons extend only as far as the door, so that he or she feels utterly abandoned and alone in the world.

When we feel bereft and alone with regard to God, when life obstructs him totally from view because of adverse circumstances, or seemingly insurmountable temptations, or illness, or depression, we think of these things as a door at the other end of the room which has been left open in readiness for his return.

The Son of Man will reappear in the heart of the individual and in the heart of the world's turmoil at some quite unexpected moment. Prayer is life lived as a continual waiting on God in patient and joyful expectation of his return.

Action

If there is a surfeit of bad news at the moment or you are encountering particular difficulties, make a point of returning to something (a painting, a book, a view) which has made you happy in the past, and experience God's love through it.

All Saints
1 November

Reading

The days are surely coming, says the Lord, when I will make a new covenant with the house of Israel and the house of Judah. It will not be like the covenant that I made with their ancestors when I took them by the hand to bring them out of the land of Egypt – a covenant that they broke, though I was their husband, says the Lord. But this is the covenant that I will make with the house of Israel after those days, says the Lord: I will put my law within them, and I will write it on their hearts; and I will be their God, and they shall be my people. No longer shall they teach one another, or say to each other, 'Know the Lord,' for they shall all know me, from the least of them to the greatest, says the Lord; for I will forgive their iniquity, and remember their sin no more (Jer. 31:31–4 NRSV).

Meditation

We are all called to be saints. It is our right and within our grasp to know and experience God fully and to be one with him. To be a saint is to desire and love God with reckless abandon and to allow his answering love to flow through us on to others. It has nothing to do with pious practices or with the dutiful attendance of church on Sundays.

Sanctity is about holy joy; joy which is unquenchable in tribulation, whole, complete and of God. It is about being abandoned to the love of God and to the love of life. Some of the most unlikely people are saints in the true sense of the word. There will be some surprises in heaven.

Christ came to be at one with us and to invite us to his party. There is a place set for each one of us at his table, a room in his house. Sanctity is not earned. It is given. All that is required of us as saints is our acceptance of the invitation to the party and our desire to be there. It is like being notified that there is a parcel waiting for collection at the main post office. The main office is Christ himself. The parcel is himself too, wholly given over to us in life as in death, now, in the times in which we live.

In the slightest inclination of the heart towards him, Christ is already there to meet us, because the love of God for the human beings of his making is beyond calculation. It exceeds the bounds of quantum physics, it is greater and more noble than the highest art form and deeper and more inscrutable than the most profound thinking. It is as good and as simple as the reconciliation of two people who have quarrelled. It is as irrepressible as the fun of playful dogs barking on a Sunday afternoon and as pure and unquestioning as a young child's acceptance of parental love.

A saint is a person who accepts without question the invitation to the party and takes rightful possession of a room in the Lord's house. Sanctity is the unquestioning acceptance of God's love.

Action

Try being a saint today, in the true sense of the word. If you find yourself happier for the experiment, try it again tomorrow and the next day, and the next . . .

Commemoration of All Souls
2 November

Reading

*Martha said to Jesus, 'Lord, if you had been here, my brother
would not have died. But even now I know that God will give you
whatever you ask of him.' Jesus said to her, 'Your brother will
rise again.' Martha said to him, 'I know that he will rise again in
the resurrection on the last day.' Jesus said to her, 'I am the
resurrection and the life. Those who believe in me, even though
they die, will live, and everyone who lives and believes in me will
never die. Do you believe this?' She said to him, 'Yes, Lord, I
believe that you are the Messiah, the Son of God, the one coming
into the world'* (John 11:21–7 NRSV).

Meditation

Christ *is* life itself, the beginning and the end, the source of all
things. He is here in the most immediate and personal way.
Christ is life today, not just at some time in the future. Martha
says that if the Lord had been there her brother would not
have died. We often think that if God had really been there,
such and such a disaster would not have happened but the
death of Christ is at the heart of every disaster and at the heart
of every disaster lies the possibility for his Resurrection and
new life to happen in the most unexpected way.

The finality of death has been cancelled in Christ's Resurrection. It has become a passing thing, a stage on a journey, a
birth into something new. We view our own physical death
much as we would view a window in an otherwise darkened

room. The constraints of earthly existence necessitate the existence of this window, not as an escape into oblivion but as a promise of the greater life and of the more brilliant light to come, once our eyes have been made strong enough for it. In allowing the pieces of ourselves which block us off from union with Christ to fall away, we strengthen the eyes of our inner being and prepare them for the brilliance of the light of the ultimate resurrection.

If someone you love has died, see yourself and them with the eyes of your heart in the company of Christ. Put yourself in Martha's position, remembering that Jesus had a great affection for Martha. Allow whatever thoughts and feelings come to you out of the reading or meditation to enfold you and the person you have lost.

Action

Visit someone who has recently been bereaved. Don't be afraid to raise the subject of their bereavement, but don't force it on them either. Be there with empathy and full attention.

Twenty-first Sunday after Trinity
Eighth before Christmas

Reading

Enter by the narrow gate; for the gate is wide and the way is easy, that leads to destruction, and those who enter by it are many. For the gate is narrow and the way is hard, that leads to life, and those who find it are few (Matt. 7:13–14).

Meditation

The kingdom of heaven, the presence of God, is come upon all of a sudden, like a scarcely trodden path leading to hidden places. The seeking of God means following this enticing path deeper and deeper into the dark mystery of the forest and farther and farther up into cloud, mist, rain and brilliant sunshine. The experience which we are called to, because prayer is a living experience of God, is both frightening and exhilarating, full of possibility and fraught with danger for 'It is a fearful thing to fall into the hands of the living God' (Heb. 10:31).

The hidden path is full of surprise encounters with aspects of ourselves that we never knew existed, both good and bad, and with knowledge radiant beyond the wildest fabrications of science fiction. It is a knowledge which is revealed in the smile of a child, in the knowing look of a cat or horse, in the shimmering beauty of new larch in spring, in all that we love most in our closest friend.

The way is hard because it is incompatible with the safety of material life devoid of spirituality. There is a choice to be made over and over again, at every turn, for no one can serve God and mammon. Once tried, the hidden path is incomparable to all the paths of the world in their predictability and tedium.

We press on madly through brambles and puddles, buffeted by branches, swept along by sudden gales of inspiration and of love for life, bogged down in difficulties, almost defeated by doubt, but always breathing the clear air of the forest and invariably coming across its Lord where we least expected to meet him.

Action

Go for a walk in the countryside, in woodland if possible, or in a park if you live in the city. Find a place where you have not walked before. If it is raining, all the better.

Twenty-second Sunday
after Trinity
Seventh before Christmas

Reading

For thus says the Lord: When seventy years are completed for Babylon, I will visit you, and I will fulfil to you my promise and bring you back to this place. For I know the plans I have for you, says the Lord, plans for welfare and not for evil, to give you a future and a hope. Then you will call upon me and come and pray to me, and I will hear you. You will seek me and find me; when you seek me with all your heart, I will be found by you, says the Lord, and I will restore your fortunes and gather you from all the nations and all the places where I have driven you, says the Lord, and I will bring you back to the place from which I sent you into exile. (Jer. 29:10–14).

Meditation

Modern life is a form of exile from our true home, for we are earthbound and out of touch with the source of life itself, ignorant of our place in the great picture of Creation. Sooner or later human beings and all living things are brought back to their beginnings, because unless a living thing dies it cannot begin again as a new being. We shall all be brought back to our beginnings, even if the process does not involve physical death.

Twenty first-century humanity will be brought back to

innocence. It will be brought back to innocence from a place of exile where there is nothing to assuage its loneliness.

Innocence does not mean ignorance. Neither is it a void of unknowing, like the void that existed before the beginning of all things. Innocence involves our being 'de-briefed' of the knowledge and desire for the things which obscure and deaden our experience of God. It is a greater knowing on a far grander scale.

Our future and our hope, as individuals and as a planet, are entirely bound up in our knowledge and experience of God. The good he has planned for us will be realised and consummated in this knowledge and experience and in the breaking down of the barriers which we have constructed for ourselves.

Action

Do anything that helps to deepen your experience of God and which loosens the bonds you may have with the things which obscure him from you. Read a good book on prayer and spirituality. Seek out a spiritual companion – everyone should have one.

Twenty-third Sunday after Trinity
Sixth before Christmas

Reading

Thus says the Lord to his anointed, to Cyrus, whose right hand I have grasped to subdue nations before him and strip kings of their robes, to open doors before him – and the gates shall not be closed: I will go before you and level the mountains, I will break in pieces the doors of bronze and cut through the bars of iron, I will give you the treasures of darkness and riches hidden in secret places, so that you may know that it is I, the Lord, the God of Israel, who call you by your name. For the sake of my servant Jacob, and Israel my chosen, I call you by your name, I surname you, though you do not know me. I am the Lord, and there is no other; besides me there is no god. I arm you, though you do not know me, so that they may know, from the rising of the sun and from the west, that there is no one besides me; I am the Lord, and there is no other. I form light and create darkness, I make weal and create woe; I the Lord do all these things. (Isa. 45:1–7).

Meditation

Spend a few minutes relaxing both inwardly and outwardly, using the method given for relaxation on pages 1 and 2. Having done this, read the passage through slowly, savouring the words and its cadence and poetry. Stay with any part of it which seems to move you particularly or speak to you in some way, without asking how it moves you or what it is saying. Just know that God is present and is speaking to you. Substitute your own name for that of Cyrus and allow the whole passage access to your heart. Leave the intellect alone for the moment. Let God speak to you in your inner darkness. Be given over from the heart. Surrender and allow your real self to be known by him, for his voice, the unspoken words in your heart, are themselves 'the treasures of darkness'.

Action

If there was anything which particularly spoke to you in this passage, if you experienced God, find a few minutes during the day to come back to that place of encounter with him. In any case, allow your heart to be revisited at odd moments during the day and during the coming week by what happened to you during the meditation.

Twenty-fourth Sunday after Trinity

Reading

Someone in the crowd said to him, 'Teacher, tell my brother to divide the family inheritance with me.' But he said to him, 'Friend, who set me to be a judge or arbitrator over you?' And he said to them, 'Take care! Be on your guard against all kinds of greed; for one's life does not consist in the abundance of possessions.' Then he told them a parable: 'The land of a rich man produced abundantly. And he thought to himself, "What should I do, for I have no place to store my crops?" Then he said, "I will do this: I will pull down my barns and build larger ones, and there I will store all my grain and my goods. And I will say to my soul, 'Soul, you have ample goods laid up for many years; relax, eat, drink, be merry.'" But God said to him, 'You fool! This very night your life is being demanded of you. And the things you have prepared, whose will they be?' So it is with those who store up treasures for themselves but are not rich toward God (Luke 12:13–21).

Meditation

We must be rich towards God, that he in turn may be rich towards us, for we have nothing which we can call our own. Material possessions and personal attributes, such as good looks and good health, intelligence and even youth, as well as talents and gifts, both spiritual and temporal, are all on loan. They are lent to us in order that we may live with them creatively as a means of fulfilment and as a source of happiness.

When a gift is hoarded and kept secret it benefits nobody, least of all the person who has the gift. What musician does not eventually tire of playing an instrument in solitude? Where is the artist who in celebrating life and all its pain and perplexity and in all its joy and transient beauty does not want to celebrate this in communion with other people? A book is only consummated when it has been read.

The privilege of living creatively, of being rich towards God in being rich towards others and towards ourselves (there is nothing sadder than people who are stingy towards themselves) consists of having something to contribute to the great wealth of human diversity and creativity which began when Adam and Eve first made marks in the sand, or cooked food, or built a shelter, or sang to one another and to the beasts.

Gifts, when used correctly, witness to God's living presence in a person. We give ourselves wholly to the present moment in allowing a little or all of the gifts we have to be taken from us, for in the present moment and in the person encountered here and now is our encounter with Christ. The more we allow to be taken from us, like a tree allowing its fruit to be picked, the more space there is in us for God to fill with his Spirit, who comes and goes like air and cannot be stifled or hidden away.

Action

Spend some time examining your gifts and being grateful for them. Look objectively at where you stand in relation to material things, to a career, a particular child, a hobby, a house. Note whether your attitude to any of these things is one of ownership and silently invite God to share in them.

Twenty-fifth Sunday after Trinity

Reading

The Lord reigns; let the peoples tremble!
He sits enthroned upon the cherubim; let the earth quake!
The Lord is great in Zion; he is exalted over all the peoples.
Let them praise thy great and terrible name! Holy is he!
Mighty King, lover of justice, thou hast established equity;
Thou hast executed justice and righteousness in Jacob.
Extol the Lord our God; worship at his footstool! Holy is he!
(Ps. 99:1–5).

Meditation

Read this passage in the context of Bethlehem. See and experience the poverty, the intimacy and the love of God brought into the lowly place of Christ's birth, who came that he might be with us and share in our human predicament in its every minute detail. 'The Lord reigns . . . He is exalted over all the peoples . . . Mighty King, lover of justice . . .' – the baby born in a stable, Emmanuel God with us.

Christ comes to bring justice into the world and to put to right the wrongs of many. He comes to bring unity out of disparate chaos, harmony and music out of sheer noise. Christ has come to enable us to put into order those things which have become disordered in ourselves and in our society, for as people grow in the knowledge and acceptance of themselves as the frail human beings that they are, they grow in awareness of the reality of the Christ-child in their lives and in the world, and in a desire to go with him in the reordering of a disordered and chaotic society.

Take into this psalm the refugee camps of the world. The Christ-child of Bethlehem has been relegated to these camps and to all the places of oppression which have been spawned in our century. He was in the streets of Soweto, on the human rubbish dumps of Mexico City, with the dispossessed Indians of the Amazon, in Sarajevo and Belfast.

Where there is conflict, where the human spirit struggles for freedom from poverty, persecution, and for the right to live in the land of their forefathers, there is Christ who for the moment has set aside his glory and majesty, the better to raise up human misery into the ultimate triumph of his kingship.

'Let the peoples tremble . . . Let the earth quake'. Let any who oppress another, who hold an individual or a nation in bondage, know that their days are numbered.

Action

Take any of these situations into your heart and respond practically. You could write a letter to a newspaper or MP, join a pressure group or take part in a peaceful demonstration.

Sunday before Advent
Fifth before Christmas

Reading

'Now concerning the times and the seasons, brothers and sisters, you do not need to have anything written to you. For you yourselves know very well that the day of the Lord will come like a thief in the night. When they say, "There is peace and security," then sudden destruction will come upon them, as labour pains come upon a pregnant woman, and there will be no escape! But you, beloved, are not in darkness, for that day to surprise you like a thief; for you are all children of light and children of the day; we are not of the night or of darkness. So then let us not fall asleep as others do, but let us keep awake and be sober; for those who sleep sleep at night, and those who are drunk get drunk at night. But since we belong to the day, let us be sober, and put on the breastplate of faith and love, and for a helmet the hope of salvation. For God has destined us not for wrath but for obtaining salvation through our Lord Jesus Christ, who died for us, so that whether we are awake or asleep we may live with him. Therefore encourage one another and build up each other as indeed you are doing' (1 Thess. 5:1–11).

Meditation

'The day of the Lord' was seen by the Jews to be a great upheaval, a purging prelude to the golden age when the world would be set to rights by the direct intervention of God. It was seen as a time of separation between the present age and the age to come.

The coming of Christ (the New Age) and his death and Resurrection are centred in the Eucharist and celebrated in the dawn of each new day and in the changing seasons. All living things serve and celebrate the birth of Christ and at the same time look forward to his return in power and great glory. We too look forward to the Parousia, the second coming, with great hope and excitement because we already know Christ in the union which we have with him heart to heart.

When the Son of Man (another word for 'ordinary man') comes again we shall greet him as one greets a loved friend who has returned to take us to a better place where the familiar things of this life have somehow been transfigured and are revealed in their true glory.

A great sadness awaits those who 'sleep' in this life and ignore the things of God, or rate them as trivial or unimportant. For the wrath of God is in fact incalculable grief for the loss of those he loves and for their rejection of him. So let us build one another up when it is hard to recognise the greatness and simplicity of his love in the superficiality and stress of another commercial Christmas.

Action

Affirm the centrality of Christ to this festival whenever you can, in conversations or preparation for Christmas.

Index of Recipes and Craft Ideas

Index of Festivals and Saints' Days